Cardiac Arrhythmias

Cardiac Arrhythmias

Practical notes on interpretation and treatment

Third Edition

David H. Bennett MD, FRCP, FACC
Consultant Cardiologist,
Regional Cardiac Centre, Wythenshawe Hospital,
Manchester

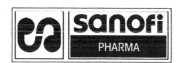
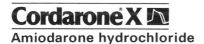
WRIGHT

London   Boston   Singapore   Sydney   Toronto   Wellington

Wright
is an imprint of Butterworth Scientific

 PART OF REED INTERNATIONAL P.L.C.

First published 1981
Second edition 1985
Reprinted 1986, 1987
Third edition 1989
Reprinted 1990

© Butterworth & Co. (Publishers) Ltd, 1989

British Library Cataloguing in Publication Data
Bennett, David H.
 Cardiac arrhythmias. - 3rd ed.
 1. Man. Heart. Arrhythmia
 I. Title
 616.1'28

 ISBN 0-7236-1595-0

Library of Congress Cataloging in Publication Data
Bennett, David H.
 Cardiac arrhythmias: practical notes on interpretation and
treatment / David H. Bennett. — 3rd ed.
  p. cm.
 Includes index.
 ISBN 0-7236-1595-0:
 1. Arrhythmia. I. Title.
 [DNLM: 1. Arrhythmia—diagnosis. 2. Arrhythmia—therapy. WG 330
B471c]
 RC685.A65B46 1989
 616.1'28—dc19
 DNLM/DLC
 for Library of Congress

Typeset by Mid-County Press, London SW15 2NW
Printed in Great Britain at the University Press, Cambridge

Preface to the third edition

The purpose of this third edition remains the same as its predecessors: to provide a practical guide to the diagnosis, investigation and management of the main cardiac arrhythmias with particular emphasis on the problems commonly encountered in practice.

Since the second edition was written some 5 years ago, there have been many developments in the understanding and management of arrhythmias. Accordingly, the text has been extensively revised and updated.

D.H.B.

Preface to the first edition

The purpose of this book is to describe the main cardiac arrhythmias, with particular emphasis on the problems commonly encountered in their interpretation, and to discuss the practical aspects of current methods of investigation and treatment. Information of purely academic value has not been included.

This book is intended to fill the gap between those textbooks that cover only the basics of arrhythmias and those that are written for the cardiac electrophysiologist. It has been written with junior hospital doctors in mind. They receive little formal training in the management of cardiac arrhythmias and yet, because prompt action is often required, the onus of diagnosis and treatment usually falls on them. It should also be of interest to medical students, who themselves will soon be responsible for dealing with arrhythmias, to nurses working in coronary and intensive care units and to physicians who want a brief review of the practical aspects of cardiac arrhythmias.

I would like to thank the cardiac technicians, coronary care nurses and medical staff at Wythenshawe Hospital for their help. I am particularly grateful to my colleagues, Dr Colin Bray and Dr Christopher Ward.

Thanks are also due to Mrs Mary Rooney for typing the manuscript and to the Wythenshawe Hospital Medical Illustration Department.

Finally, I would like to acknowledge the distractions provided by my family, Irene, Samantha and Sally, to whom this book is dedicated.

D.H.B.

Contents

Notes

Unless otherwise indicated, the electrocardiograms in this book have been recorded at a paper speed of 25 mm/s. At this speed, each large square represents 0·2 s and each small square represents 0·04 s.

Heart rate (beats/minute) can be calculated by dividing the number of large squares between two consecutive complexes into 300, or by dividing the number of small squares between two complexes into 1500.

To include the relevant features in the electrocardiograms, some records have had to be reduced in size.

When assessing a cardiac rhythm it should be remembered that only atrial and ventricular activity register on the surface electrocardiogram. The site of impulse formation, sequence of cardiac chamber activation and functions of the sinus node and atrioventricular junction have to be deduced from analysis of the atrial and ventricular electrograms. A single 'rhythm strip' may be inadequate for diagnosis. Scrutiny of several ECG leads, preferably recorded simultaneously, may be necessary. For example, atrial activity is often the key to diagnosis but may not be clearly shown in all ECG leads: it is often best seen in leads II and V1.

An electrocardiogram of an arrhythmia that is of diagnostic importance or that leads to the initiation of or a change in treatment should always be recorded and safely stored. This guideline which may be relevant to the long-term management of a patient (e.g. pacemaker implantation or antiarrhythmic therapy) is not infrequently ignored, particularly on intensive care units!

Chapter 1

Sinus rhythm

The sinus node is the primary pacemaker of the heart, initiating the electrical activity that leads to the orderly activation of atrial and then ventricular myocardium during each heart beat. Sinus node activity does not register on the electrocardiogram (ECG).

Atrial activity, the P wave, can be seen in most ECG leads (Figure 1.1). Sometimes the P wave is of low amplitude and it may be necessary to inspect all leads of the ECG to establish that the patient is in sinus rhythm (Figure 1.2).

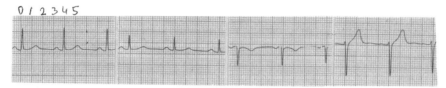

Figure 1.1 Sinus rhythm (leads I, AVR, AVR and V2). Atrial activity is clearly seen in the limb leads but is only just discernible in V2

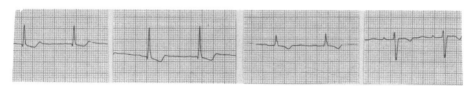

Figure 1.2 Sinus rhythm with low-amplitude P waves (leads I, II, III and V1). Atrial activity is only clearly seen in V1

Atrial activation spreads from the sinus node, which lies at the junction of the superior vena cava and right atrium, in an inferior direction. The P wave, therefore, is upright in leads II, III and AVF, which are orientated towards the inferior surface of the heart, and is inverted in AVR, which is orientated towards the superior heart surface (Figure 1.1). If the P wave does not have these characteristics then, even though each ventricular complex is preceded by a P wave, the rhythm is abnormal (Figure 1.3).

The atrioventricular (AV) node delays the transmission of the activating impulse from atria to ventricles. This is reflected by the PR interval, which is measured from

1

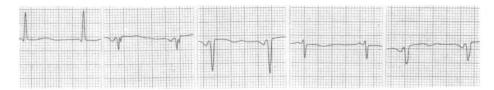

Figure 1.3 Junctional rhythm (leads I, II, III, AVR, AVF): a P wave precedes each QRS complex but is superiorly directed

the onset of the P wave to the onset of the ventricular complex. The normal PR interval ranges from 0·12 to 0·21 s. It shortens with increasing heart rate.

After traversing the AV node, the electrical impulse is conducted very rapidly by the bundle of His and right and left bundle branches to the ventricular myocardium. Ventricular activation is represented by the QRS complex which, in the absence of bundle branch block, should be less than 0·08 s in duration.

The characteristics of normal sinus rhythm

P wave

- Precedes each QRS complex
- Upright in leads III, AVF
- Inverted in lead AVR

PR interval
- Duration 0·12–0·21 s

QRS complex
- Duration less than 0·08 s

Sinus bradycardia

This is defined as sinus rhythm at a rate less then 60/min (Figure 1.4). It may be physiological, as in athletes, or caused by acute myocardial infarction, sick sinus syndrome or beta-adrenoceptor blocking drugs. Non-cardiac disorders such as myxoedema, jaundice and raised intracranial pressure can also cause sinus bradycardia.

The rate may be increased by atropine or by pacing but treatment is only indicated in circumstances when sinus bradycardia causes symptoms, tachyarrhythmia or marked hypotension.

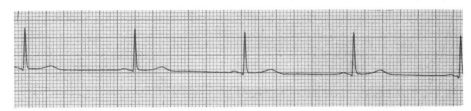

Figure 1.4 Sinus bradycardia. Rate is 48/min

Sinus tachycardia

This is defined as sinus rhythm at a rate greater than 100/min (Figure 1.5). Sinus tachycardia is caused by exercise, anxiety or any disorder that increases sympathetic nervous system activity. Occasionally it may be due to a primary disorder of the sinus node (sinus node re-entry).

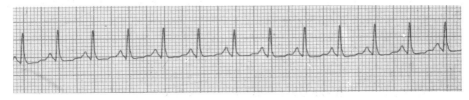

Figure 1.5 Sinus tachycardia during exercise (lead II). The rate is 150/min

Sinus tachycardia is usually a physiological response and as such does not require specific treatment. However, if sinus tachycardia is inappropriate, the rate may be slowed by beta-adrenoceptor blocking drugs.

At rest the sinus node rate is seldom above 120/min unless the patient is very ill. In contrast, atrial flutter with 2:1 AV block often leads to a heart rate of 140–160/min and can easily be mistaken for sinus tachycardia (see Chapter 6).

Sinus arrhythmia

Normally there are only minor changes in rate during sinus rhythm. In sinus arrhythmia there are alternating periods of slowing and increasing sinus node rate. Usually the rate increases during inspiration (Figure 1.6). Sinus arrhythmia is most commonly seen in the young.

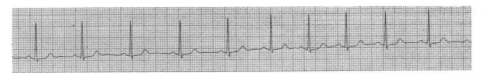

Figure 1.6 Sinus arrhythmia

Main points

- For sinus rhythm, an inferiorly directed P wave (i.e. upright in leads III and AVF) must precede each QRS complex.

- If AV conduction is normal, the duration of the PR interval will be between 0·12 and 0·21 s.

- Normal intraventricular conduction results in a QRS complex whose duration will be less than 0·08 s.

- In cases of apparent sinus tachycardia at rest, atrial flutter or tachycardia should be excluded.

Chapter 2

Ectopic beats

The terms ectopic beat, extrasystole and premature contraction differ in their precise meanings but are, for practical purposes, synonymous. They refer to an impulse originating from the atria, AV junction (i.e. AV node plus Bundle of His) or ventricles, which arises prematurely in the cardiac cycle (Figures 2.1–2.3).

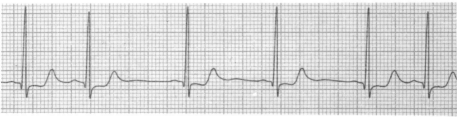

Figure 2.1 Atrial ectopic beats (second and sixth beats). The ectopic P waves differ slightly in shape from those of sinus origin

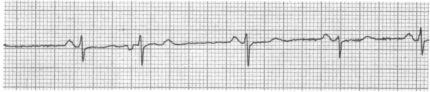

Figure 2.2 The second beat is a junctional ectopic beat (lead III). The junctional focus has activated the atria as well as the ventricles, resulting in an inverted P wave which precedes the QRS complex

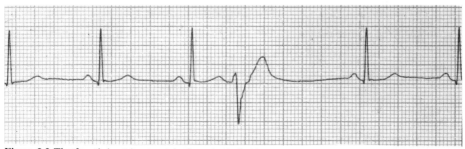

Figure 2.3 The fourth beat is a ventricular ectopic beat

Ectopic beats are premature. Thus the interval between the ectopic beat and the preceding beat (i.e. the coupling interval) is always shorter than the cycle length of the dominant rhythm. This fact is often forgotten, with the result that other beats with abnormal configurations, i.e. escape beats (see Chapter 3) and intermittent bundle branch block (see Chapter 4), are misinterpreted as ectopic beats. Whereas suppression of ectopic beats may be desirable, attempts to suppress escape beats and beats with bundle branch block can be dangerous.

Usually, ectopic beats arising from the same focus have the same coupling interval and configuration (Figure 2.4).

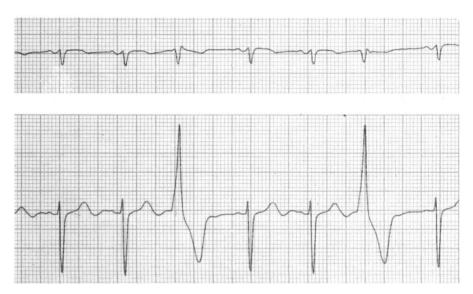

Figure 2.4 Simultaneous recording of leads V1 and V2. The third and sixth beats are unifocal ventricular ectopic beats. Their ventricular origin is not apparent in lead V1 but is obvious in V2

The site of origin of an ectopic beat can be ascertained from careful examination of the ECG. It cannot be stressed too strongly that a single rhythm strip does not always reveal the diagnostic clues and that scrutiny of simultaneous recordings of several ECG leads is often necessary (Figures 2.4 and 2.5).

Atrial ectopic beats

These are recognized by a P wave which is premature and, because the source and hence direction of atrial activation differ from that during sinus rhythm, these P waves will often be of abnormal shape (see Figure 2.1). Ectopic P waves may be smaller than normal, and because they are premature they may be superimposed on the T wave of the preceding beat. Careful examination of the ECG is essential to detect ectopic P waves; frequently they are best shown in lead V1 (Figures 2.5 and 2.6).

Usually an atrial ectopic beat will be conducted to the ventricles in the same manner as if the atria had been activated by the sinus node. Thus the PR interval and QRS complex of the ectopic beat will be identical with those during sinus rhythm

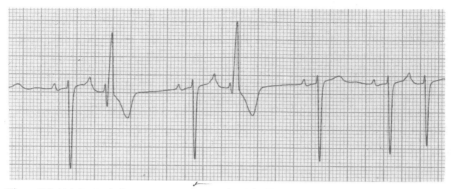

Figure 2.5 Atrial ectopic beats are superimposed on the T waves of the first, third and sixth ventricular complexes (lead V1). It can be seen how the T waves of these beats are modified by comparing them with the T wave of the fifth ventricular complex which is not followed by an atrial ectopic. The first two atrial ectopic beats are aberrantly conducted, resulting in right bundle branch block

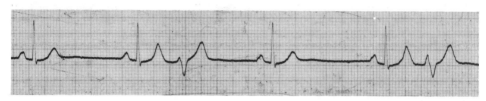

Figure 2.6 The third and sixth beats are atrial ectopic beats. The premature P waves are superimposed on the preceding T wave, as can be seen by comparing the T waves of sinus beats preceding and not preceding ectopic beats. The ectopic beats show first-degree AV block and phasic aberrant conduction

(see Figure 2.1). If the QRS complex during sinus rhythm shows bundle branch block, then so will the QRS complex in the ectopic beat.

Sometimes, however, atrial ectopic beats, especially those that arise very early in the cardiac cycle, may encounter either an AV junction or bundle branch which has not yet recovered from conduction of the last atrial impulse and is, therefore, partially or completely refractory to excitation. Partial and complete refractoriness of the AV junction will result in prolongation of the PR interval and blocked atrial ectopic beats, respectively (Figures 2.6–2.8). Blocked atrial ectopics have on occasion

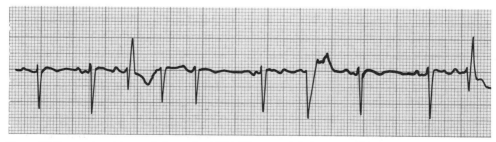

Figure 2.7 Frequent atrial ectopic beats (lead V1). The seventh beat is an atrial ectopic beat conducted with left bundle branch block and marked prolongation of the PR interval. The third and tenth beats are atrial ectopic beats conducted with right bundle branch block and slight prolongation of the PR interval

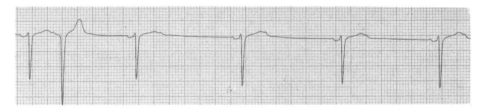

Figure 2.8 Atrial ectopic beats are superimposed on the T wave of each ventricular complex. The first atrial ectopic is conducted with partial left branch block. The other atrial ectopic beats are not conducted to the ventricles

been erroneously taken as an indication for cardiac pacing! Partial or complete refractoriness of one or other bundle branch (it is usually the right bundle) will lead to correspondingly partial or complete bundle branch block (Figure 2.7). This phenomenon of functional bundle branch block is referred to as 'phasic aberrant intraventricular conduction'. The practical significance of this phenomenon is that the resultant QRS complexes are broad and can therefore mimic ventricular ectopic beats.

The characteristics of atrial ectopic beats. The P wave:

- Will be premature
- May be superimposed on and distort the preceding T wave
- Usually, followed by normal QRS complex
- Sometimes, results in AV or bundle branch block

Clinical significance of atrial ectopic beats

Atrial ectopic beats are often benign. However, if they are frequent they may mimic atrial fibrillation and may herald its onset. When frequent atrial ectopic beats occur in patients with heart disease, especially valve disorders, myocardial infarction, cardiomyopathy or following cardiac surgery, treatment with digoxin should be considered so that the ventricular rate will be controlled should atrial fibrillation occur.

AV junctional ectopic beats

AV junctional beats used to be referred to as 'nodal' beats. It is now appreciated that at least part of the AV node is not capable of pacemaker activity and that it is not possible to distinguish between beats of AV nodal and His bundle origin. Hence the more general term 'AV junction'.

AV junctional ectopic beats are recognized by a premature QRS complex similar to that occurring in sinus rhythm. The atria as well as the ventricles may be activated by the junctional focus, leading to an inverted P wave (i.e. negative in leads II, III and AVF) which may precede, follow or be buried within the QRS complex, depending on the relative speeds of conduction from AV junction to ventricles and from AV junction to atria (see Figure 2.2).

AV junctional ectopic beats are not as common as atrial or ventricular ectopics. Treatment is rarely required.

Ventricular ectopic beats

These are recognized by a premature ventricular complex which is broad (usually >0·12 s), bizarre in shape and, in contrast to atrial ectopic beats, will clearly not be preceded by an ectopic P wave (see Figures 2.3 and 2.4). The abnormal shape and prolonged duration of the ventricular complex reflect the abnormal course and consequent slowing of ventricular activation.

In ventricular ectopic beats the QRS complex will:

- Be premature
- Be broad (>0·12 s)
- Be abnormal in shape
- Not be preceded by a premature P wave

A number of different terms are used to describe ventricular ectopic beats, as follows.

Unifocal or multifocal

Ectopic beats with the same shape and coupling intervals are assumed to arise from the same focus, whereas differing contours and coupling intervals imply more than one focus (see Figures 2.4 and 2.9).

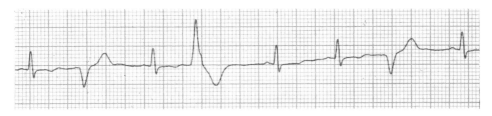

Figure 2.9 Multifocal ventricular ectopic beats. The second ventricular ectopic beat has a different shape and coupling interval from the first and third ectopic beats

Early ventricular ectopic beats

Ectopic beats that occur very early in the cardiac cycle will be superimposed on the T wave of the preceding beat and are described as 'R on T' (Figure 2.10). Most

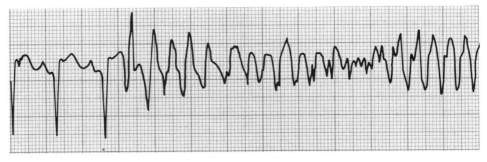

Figure 2.10 An 'R on T' ventricular ectopic beat initiates ventricular fibrillation

episodes of ventricular fibrillation and many episodes of ventricular tachycardia are initiated by 'R on T' ectopics (though by no means do all 'R on T' ectopic beats precipitate these arrhythmias).

Late ventricular ectopic beats

A ventricular ectopic beat that occurs late in the cardiac cycle may fall, by chance, immediately after a P wave initiated by sinus node activity (the P wave will therefore be normal in timing and configuration). This is referred to as an 'end-diastolic' ventricular ectopic beat (Figure 2.11). This situation, in which the atrial impulse will clearly not be conducted to the ventricles, must not be confused with an ectopic atrial beat with aberrant conduction – in which case, of course, the P wave will be premature.

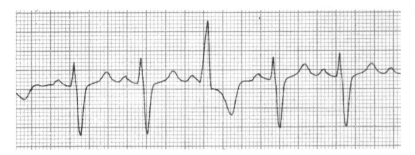

Figure 2.11 The third beat is an end-diastolic ventricular ectopic beat. It is preceded by a *normally* timed P wave

Because the initial upstroke of a ventricular ectopic beat may be slurred like a delta wave (see Chapter 7), end-diastolic ventricular ectopic beats can mimic the Wolff–Parkinson–White syndrome (Figure 2.12).

Interpolated ventricular ectopic beats

Usually there is a pause after a ventricular ectopic beat before the next beat. When there is no such pause and the ectopic beat is thus sandwiched between two normal beats, the ectopic beat is said to be 'interpolated' (Figure 2.13).

Frequency

Ventricular ectopic beats are usually quantified in terms of the number occurring per minute.

When an ectopic beat follows each sinus beat the term bigeminy is applied (Figure 2.14). If an ectopic follows a pair of normal beats there is trigeminy. When two ectopics occur in succession (Figure 2.15) they are referred to as a couplet, and when there are more than two ectopic beats in succession the group is termed a salvo or ventricular tachycardia (see Chapter 5).

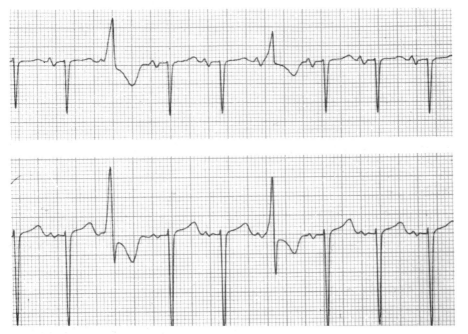

Figure 2.12 Simultaneous recording of leads V1 and V2. Two end-diastolic ventricular ectopic beats. The second mimicking the Wolff–Parkinson–White syndrome

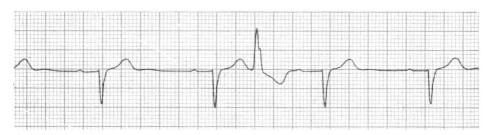

Figure 2.13 Interpolated ventricular beat. The subsequent PR interval is prolonged owing to retrograde concealed conduction

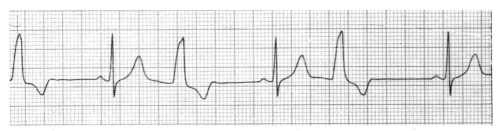

Figure 2.14 Ventricular bigeminy

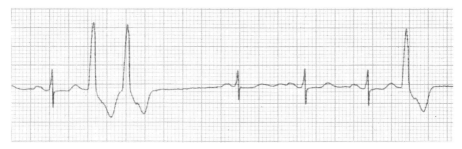

Figure 2.15 The first sinus beat is followed by a couplet of ventricular ectopic beats

Atrial activity

The pattern of atrial activity following a ventricular ectopic beat depends on whether the AV junction transmits the ventricular impulse back to the atria. If this occurs the result is an inverted P wave which is often superimposed on and may be concealed by the ventricular ectopic beat (Figure 2.16).

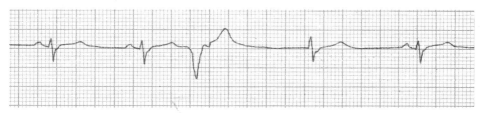

Figure 2.16 The third beat is a ventricular ectopic beat which has been conducted back to the atria, resulting in an inverted P wave (lead AVF). The ectopic beat is followed by a junctional escape beat

When the AV junction does not transmit the ventricular impulse to the atria, atrial activity proceeds independently of ventriculr activity; it is only in these cases that a ventricular impulse will be followed by a full compensatory pause, i.e. the lengths of the cycles before and after the ectopic beat will equal twice the sinus cycle length (see Figures 2.3 and 2.4).

Sometimes a ventricular impulse only partially penetrates the AV junction. Particularly with interpolated ventricular ectopics, the subsequent atrial impulse arising from sinus node activation may find the AV junction partially refractory and be conducted with a prolonged PR interval (Figure 2.13). The significance of this phenomenon of 'retrograde concealed conduction' is that the prolonged PR interval in these circumstances does not indicate AV node disease, and if the phenomenon is observed in first beat after a tachycardia, a ventricular origin for the tachycardia can be inferred (see Chapter 8).

Parasystole

As stated above, unifocal ventricular ectopic beats have a constant coupling interval. Ventricular parasystole, a rare phenomenon, is an exception to this rule. In this arrhythmia a ventricular ectopic focus discharges regularly, undisturbed by the dominant rhythm, and will capture the ventricles provided that the ectopic discharge

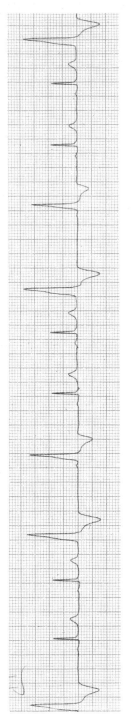

Figure 2.17 Ventricular parasystole. The ectopic beats have a variable coupling interval. The intervals between ectopic beats are multiples of 1·18 s. The fifth and ninth beats are fusion beats

does not occur when the ventricles have just been activated by the dominant rhythm and are therefore refractory.

Thus ventricular parasystole (Figure 2.17) is characterized by a variable coupling interval, inter-ectopic intervals which are multiples of a common factor and, because the ventricles may by chance be simultaneously activated by both ectopic and normal pacemakers, fusion beats (complexes that in appearance are a fusion between normal and ectopic beats).

Causes of ventricular ectopic beats

Causes include acute myocardial ischaemia and infarction, chronic ischaemic heart disease, myocarditis, cardiomyopathies, mitral valve prolapse, valvular heart disease and digoxin toxicity. Not infrequently, no cause is found.

Exercise ECG testing, echocardiography and ambulatory electrocardiography should be considered in the assessment of the patient.

Significance of ventricular ectopic beats

Occasional ventricular ectopic beats at rest and even frequent unifocal ectopic beats on exercise occur in otherwise normal individuals and are not necessarily pathological or of prognostic significance.

In contrast, 'complex' ventricular ectopic beats – i.e. frequent, multifocal, 'R on T' or those that occur in salvoes – are rarely found in the absence of cardiac disease and are associated with an increased cardiovascular mortality. In the setting of chronic ischaemic heart disease, a correlation between severity of left ventricular damage and frequency of ectopic beats has been demonstrated. Recent evidence, however, points to the presence of ectopic beats as an additional and independent risk factor. At present, there is no hard evidence to show that suppression or reduction in frequency of ectopic beats by anti-arrhythmic therapy improves prognosis.

Whereas ectopic beats in many individuals are asymptomatic, they may cause distressing symptoms in others, including those without evidence of structural heart disease. Symptomatic patients may be distressed by the irregularity caused by premature beats, the compensatory pause and/or 'thump' caused by increased myocardial contractility associated with the post-ectopic beat. In this minority of patients anti-arrhythmic therapy may be indicated for purely symptomatic purposes.

The significance of ventricular ectopic beats in acute myocardial infarction is discussed in Chapter 11.

Main points

- Ectopic beats are premature and therefore have a coupling interval shorter than the cycle length of the dominant rhythm.

- The P waves of atrial ectopic beats are often superimposed on the preceding T wave and can easily be missed. They are usually best seen in lead V1.

- Atrial ectopic beats may cause partial or complete AV or bundle branch block.

- Ventricular ectopic beats cause premature, broad and bizarrely shaped QRS complexes. They are only followed by a full compensatory pause if they are not conducted to the atria.

- Chronic ventricular ectopic beats which are frequent, multifocal, 'R on T' or occur in salvoes are associated with an increased cardiovascular mortality but there is little evidence to show that their suppression improves prognosis.

Chapter 3

Escape beats

Escape beats arise from subsidiary pacemaker tissue when the dominant pacemaker fails to discharge. In contrast to ectopic beats, they are always late, i.e. the coupling interval is greater than the cycle length of the dominant rhythm (Figures 3.1 and 3.3). Distinction between escape and ectopic beats is important because the former should clearly not be suppressed by drugs.

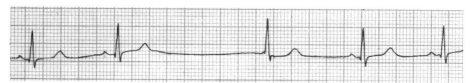

Figure 3.1 The third ventricular complex is a junctional escape beat. By chance, it is superimposed on a P wave which occurs too late to capture the ventricles

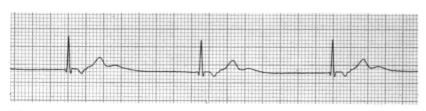

Figure 3.2 Junctional escape rhythm (lead II). The junctional focus has activated the atria as indicated by the inverted P wave following each QRS complex

Escape beats are usually of junctional origin (Figures 3.1–3.3). Less commonly, they arise from the ventricles. The ventricular complexes of junctional escape beats are similar to those during normal rhythm. Ventricular escape beats have a similar configuration to ventricular ectopic beats (Figure 3.4).

Escape beats themselves require no treatment. If treatment is indicated, it is to accelerate the basic rhythm.

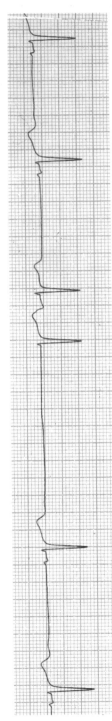

Figure 3.3 The third ventricular complex is a junctional escape beat which arises after a period of sinus arrest. The escape beat is followed by an atrial ectopic beat which is superimposed on the preceding T wave and is conducted with a prolonged PR interval

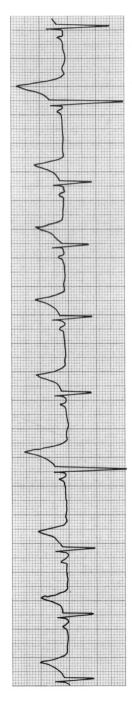

Figure 3.4 The fourth and ninth ventricular complexes are escape beats, probably arising from the ventricles, which result from slowing of the sinus node rate. P waves precede the escape beats but they are unlikely to have captured the ventricles since the PR intervals are shorter than during sinus rhythm

Main points

- The coupling interval of escape beats is greater than the cycle length of the dominant rhythm.

- As with ectopic beats, the configuration of escape beats indicates whether they are of supraventricular or ventricular origin.

- In contrast to ectopic beats, suppression of escape beats by drugs should not be attempted.

Chapter 4

Bundle branch blocks

The bundle of His divides into left and right bundle branches. The left bundle branch has two main subdivisions: the anterior and posterior fascicles.

Right bundle branch block

In right bundle branch block, activation of the right ventricle is delayed. Septal and left ventricular activation are unaffected.

Delayed right ventricular activation is reflected by an increase in duration of the QRS complex ($\geqslant$0·12 s), a secondary R wave in leads orientated to the right ventricle (V1 and V2) and a slurred S wave in left ventricular leads, especially lead I (Figure 4.1).

Partial right bundle branch block gives rise to a similar ECG appearance but the QRS duration is 0·11 s or less.

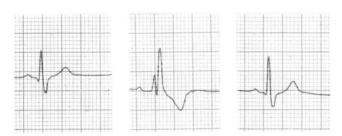

Figure 4.1 Right bundle branch block (leads I, V1, V6). There is an M-shaped complex in V1 and a deep slurred S wave in leads I and V6

Causes

Right bundle branch block may be an isolated congenital lesion. It is often found in congenital heart disease and other causes of right ventricular hypertrophy or strain.

Right bundle branch block is common when there is disease of the specialized conducting tissues. Phasic aberrant intraventricular conduction may cause intermittent right bundle branch block.

Based on limited data, neither pre-existing or acquired right bundle branch block appear to be of poor prognostic significance.

Left bundle branch block

In left bundle branch block, activation of the interventricular septum is initiated by impulses arising from the right bundle branch and is therefore in the opposite direction to normal. Thus the initial small negative (q) wave normally seen in left ventricular leads (V5, V6, I and AVL) is replaced by a larger positive (R) wave. Activation of the left ventricle will be delayed and this results in a secondary R wave in left ventricular leads and prolongation of the duration of the QRS complex ($\geqslant 0.12$ s). The primary and secondary R waves produce an M-shaped ventricular complex in left ventricular leads (Figure 4.2). In contrast, right bundle branch block produces an M-shaped ventricular complex in right ventricular leads.

Partial left bundle branch block has a similar ECG appearance to complete left bundle branch block, but the QRS duration is 0·10 or 0·11 s.

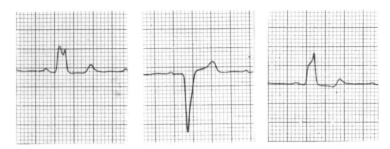

Figure 4.2 Left bundle branch block (leads I, V1, V6). There is an M-shaped complex in I and V6. The QS complex in V1 is also characteristic of left bundle branch block

Causes

Causes include coronary artery disease, severe left ventricular hypertrophy and cardiomyopathy. Rarely, left bundle branch block may occur in an otherwise normal heart.

Like right bundle branch block, left bundle branch block can be due to disease of the specialized conduction tissues. It can also occur as a result of phasic aberrant intraventricular conduction. Left bundle branch block can be intermittent (Figure 4.3).

The finding of recently acquired left bundle branch block indicates that the patient is at a substantially increased risk of sudden death.

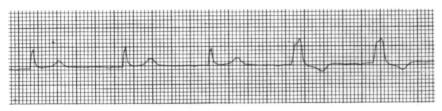

Figure 4.3 Intermittent left bundle branch block (lead AVL)

Left anterior and posterior fascicular blocks

The anterior and posterior fascicles of the left bundle branch conduct impulses to the anterosuperior and posteroinferior regions of the left ventricle, respectively.

Block can occur in either the anterior or posterior fascicle and is known as fascicular block or hemiblock. Explanation of the diagnosis of the fascicular blocks is based on the hexaxial reference system.

Hexaxial reference system

Whereas the chest leads reflect electrical activity in the horizontal plane, the limb leads reflect activity in the frontal plane. The hexaxial reference system is a method of displaying the orientation of the six limb leads to the heart in the frontal plane (Figure 4.4).

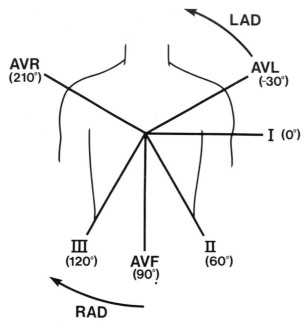

Figure 4.4 Hexaxial reference system. LAD, left axis deviation; RAD, right axis deviation

For example, a superiorly directed impulse will move away from leads II, III and AVF, producing a negative wave in these leads, and towards AVL, producing a positive wave in this lead.

The direction of an impulse can be expressed in terms of the number of degrees clockwise (positive) or anticlockwise (negative) of lead I, which is the zero reference point. For example, an impulse directed towards lead AVL has an axis of $-30°$ and an impulse directed towards lead III has an axis of $+120°$ (Figure 4.4).

Mean frontal QRS axis

The mean frontal QRS axial describes the dominant or average direction of the various electrical forces that develop during ventricular activation. Normally, the mean frontal QRS axis lies between AVL (i.e. −30°) and AVF (i.e. +90°). If the axis is counterclockwise, or to the left of AVL (i.e. less than −30°), it is termed abnormal left axis deviation. If the axis is clockwise, or to the right of AVF (i.e. more than +90°), there is right axis deviation.

Using the hexaxial reference system, the mean frontal QRS axis may be calculated to within a few degrees. From the practical point of view, however, this degree of precision is unnecessary. Furthermore, though the method for calculating the axis is straightforward, errors are often made, sometimes leading to inappropriate action, e.g. unnecessary pacemaker insertion. It is easier and quite proper to diagnose left and right axis deviation from a simple rule of thumb, as follows.

In left axis deviation, lead I is predominantly positive and both leads II and III are predominantly negative (Figure 4.5). Contrary to some older texts, *both* II and III must be predominantly negative, i.e. if in lead II the S wave is smaller than the R wave, left axis deviation is not present (Figure 4.6). If lead II is equiphasic, there is borderline left axis deviation (Figure 4.6). In right axis deviation lead I is predominantly negative and both leads II and III are predominantly positive (Figure 4.7).

Left anterior fascicular block

Block in the anterior fascicle of the left bundle branch causes delay in activation of the anterosuperior portion of the left ventricle, whilst activation of the posteroinferior portion is unaffected.

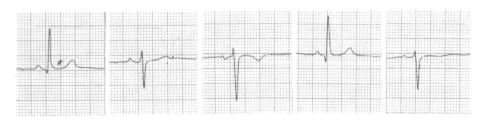

Figure 4.5 Left axis deviation due to left anterior fascicular block (leads I, II, III, AVL, AVF)

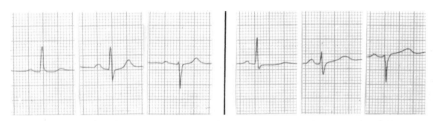

Figure 4.6 Leads I, II, III from two patients. In the first, the mean frontal QRS axis is normal. In the second, lead II is equiphasic and thus there is borderline left axis deviation

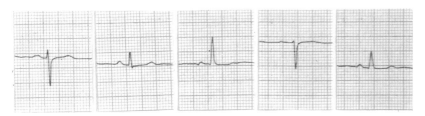

Figure 4.7 Right axis deviation due to left posterior fascicular block (leads I, II, III, AVL, AVF)

Initial left ventricular activation will be via the posterior fascicle to the postero-inferior region and will therefore be directed inferiorly and to the right. This results in an initial positive deflection (r wave) in inferiorly orientated leads (II, III and AVF) and in an initial negative deflection (q wave) in the lateral leads (I and AVL) (see Figure 4.5).

The anterosuperior region will be activated by conduction from the posteroinferior region. The resultant wave will, therefore, be superiorly directed (R wave in I and AVL; S in II, III and AVF). Because conduction is through ordinary myocardium rather than the specialized conducting tissues, it will be relatively slow. As a result, activation of the anterosuperior region will be delayed and consequently unopposed by activity from the rest of the ventricles. Thus the resultant superiorly directed wave is larger than the initial inferiorly directed wave and the mean frontal QRS axis will also be superiorly directed, i.e. there will be left axis deviation.

Left anterior fascicular block is a common cause of left axis deviation. There are other causes, however; inferior myocardial infarction (Figure 4.8) for example. To diagnose left anterior fascicular block two criteria must be satisfied. First, there must be left axis deviation, i.e. lead I must be predominantly positive and leads II and III predominantly negative. Secondly, the initial direction of ventricular activation must be inferior and to the right, i.e. there must be an initial r wave in leads II, III and AVF.

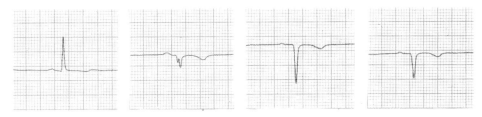

Figure 4.8 Inferior myocardial infarction (leads I, II, III, AVF). There is left axis deviation but not left anterior fascicular block

Left posterior fascicular block

In left posterior fascicular block activation of the posteroinferior portion of the left ventricle is delayed. As a result, there will be an initial positive (r) wave in leads I and AVL and an initial negative (q) wave in leads II, III and AVF; and there will be right axis deviation, i.e. lead I will be predominantly negative and leads II and III predominantly positive (see Figure 4.7).

A diagnosis of left posterior fascicular block can only be made in the absence of other causes of right axis deviation, i.e. any cause of right ventricular hypertrophy or strain, or a young patient with an asthenic build.

Left anterior and posterior fascicular blocks are commonly seen in conduction tissue disease. Their significance is discussed in Chapter 9.

Main points

♦ Complete bundle branch block prolongs QRS duration to 0·12 s or greater. In incomplete block QRS duration is 0·10–0·11 s.

♦ In left axis deviation, lead I is predominantly positive and leads II and III are predominantly negative.

♦ In right axis deviation, lead I is predominantly negative and leads II and III positive.

♦ The criteria for left anterior hemiblock are left axis deviation together with a small, initial r wave in leads II and AVF.

♦ Left posterior hemiblock should be considered when there is right axis deviation in the absence of its other causes, e.g. right ventricular hypertrophy or strain.

Chapter 5

Ventricular tachycardia

Ventricular tachycardia is defined as three or more ventricular ectopic beats in rapid succession. The rate is usually between 120 and 250 beats per minute. A similar rhythm with a rate below 120 beats per minute is termed accelerated idioventricular rhythm (see below).

The arrhythmia may cause shock, cardiac arrest or progress to ventricular fibrillation. On the other hand, in some circumstances it may be well tolerated with few or no symptoms.

The main causes of ventricular tachycardia

- Acute myocardial ischaemia or infarction
- Chronic ischaemic heart disease
- Dilated cardiomyopathy
- Hypertrophic cardiomyopathy
- Myocarditis
- Right ventricular dysplasia
- Mitral valve prolapse
- Valvular heart disease
- Drug toxicity, e.g. digoxin, quinidine
- Cardiac surgery
- Idiopathic

There are three types of ventricular tachycardia:

1. Monomorphic ventricular tachycardia.
2. Accelerated idioventricular rhythm.
3. Polymorphic ventricular tachycardia.

Monomorphic ventricular tachycardia

This is the commonest form of ventricular tachycardia.

ECG characteristics

It consists of a rapid succession of ventricular ectopic beats of uniform appearance (Figures 5.1–5.3). Each complex will thus be abnormal in shape, and the duration of each complex will be in excess of 0·12 s and often greater than 0·14 s. The rhythm is

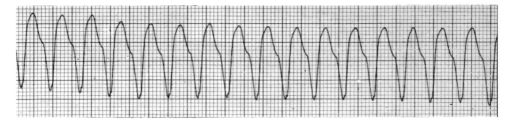

Figure 5.1 Ventricular tachycardia. The complexes are broad and bizarre. The rhythm is regular

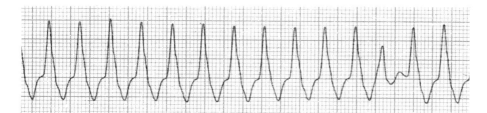

Figure 5.2 Ventricular tachycardia (lead V1). The twelfth complex is a fusion beat

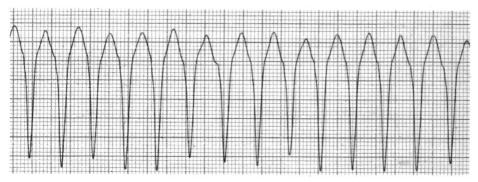

Figure 5.3 Ventricular tachycardia (lead V1)

regular unless there are capture beats (see below) which cause minor irregularities in the rhythm.

The characteristics of monomorphic ventricular tachycardia

- Rate of 120–250 beats per minute
- Regular rhythm
- Broad (>0·12 s) complexes
- Uniform complexes
- Independent P wave often present
- Capture or fusion beats often present

Atrial activity during ventricular tachycardia
In many ventricular tachycardias atrial activity continues to be initiated by the sinus

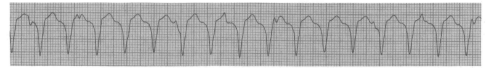

Figure 5.4 Ventricular tachycardia with direct evidence of independent atrial activity. P waves, separated by intervals of 0.75 s, can be seen after the 1st, 3rd, 6th, 8th, 10th, 13th, 15th and 17th ventricular complexes

node and therefore proceeds independently of, and at a slower rate than, ventricular activity (Figure 5.4). In others, the ventricular impulses are conducted via the AV junction to the atria so that each ventricular complex is followed by an inverted P wave (rarely second-degree block may occur in the AV junction so that only a proportion of ventricular impulses are conducted to the atria). Usually the retrograde P wave is concealed by the superimposed terminal portion of the ventricular complex (Figure 5.5).

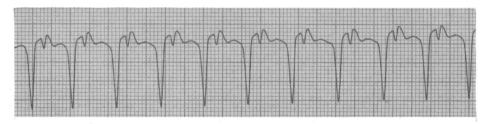

Figure 5.5 Ventricular tachycardia (lead AVF) with retrograde atrial activation. Each ventricular complex can be seen to be followed by an inverted P wave

Identification of independent atrial activity during a tachycardia excludes an origin at AV node level or above and is thus an important pointer towards ventricular tachycardia rather than supraventricular tachycardia with bundle branch block (aberrant conduction). There may be direct or indirect evidence of independent atrial activity.

Direct evidence of independent atrial activity
Direct evidence of independent atrial activity wll be demonstrated by P waves inscribed at a slower rate than and dissociated from ventricular activity (Figure 5.4). Inevitably, some P waves will be concealed by superimposed ventricular complexes. Furthermore, not all leads will clearly show atrial activity: a rhythm strip is often inadequate and scrutiny of a simultaneous recording of several different leads may be necessary. Sometimes there will be doubt as to whether small waves found on the ECG during tachycardia are actually caused by atrial activity. If they are, they will be separated by similar intervals, or multiples of that interval.

Indirect evidence of independent atrial activity
Capture or fusion beats are indirect evidence of atrial activity. The finding of just one of these beats is sufficient to exclude an origin for the tachycardia above the level of the AV junction.

Capture beats occur when the timing of an atrial impulse during ventricular tachycardia is such that it can be transmitted via the AV junction and activate the ventricles before the next discharge from the ventricular focus. This results in a normal and therefore narrower ventricular complex occurring slightly earlier than the next ventricular ectopic beat would be expected (Figure 5.6).

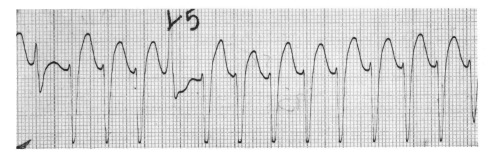

Figure 5.6 Ventricular tachycardia (lead V5). The 'fifth' complex is a capture beat and the first complex is a fusion beat

Fusion beats are caused by a similar process. However, the atrial impulse activates the ventricles slightly later in the cardiac cycle leading to simultaneous activation of the ventricles by the transmitted atrial impulse and the ventricular ectopic focus. The result is a ventricular complex which in appearance is a fusion between a normal QRS complex and a ventricular ectopic beat (see Figures 5.2, 5.6 and 5.7).

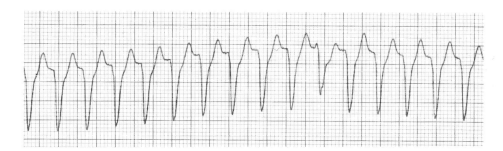

Figure 5.7 Ventricular tachycardia. The eleventh complex is a fusion beat

Fascicular tachycardia

This is a rare monomorphic ventricular tachycardia thought to arise from the posterior fascicle of the left bundle branch and is not associated with structural heart disease. It is characterized by ventricular complexes which are relatively short (0·12 s) in duration with the configuration of right bundle branch block and left axis deviation (Figure 5.8).

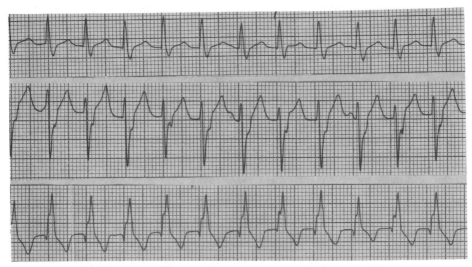

Figure 5.8 Fascicular tachycardia (leads I, II, and V1). Independent atrial activity can be seen in lead II

Management of monomorphic ventricular tachycardia

Choice of treatment depends on:

1. The degree of circulatory disturbance.
2. Whether the arrhythmia is likely to recur.
3. The prognosis.

Ventricular tachycardia that is not due to an acute event such as acute myocardial infarction or drug toxicity is very likely to recur sooner or later. When the arrhythmia is associated with significant structural heart disease and/or has caused marked hypotension or shock, the prognosis without treatment is poor.

Termination of tachycardia
Options include cardioversion, drugs, pacing and electrical stimulation.

Cardioversion
If sustained ventricular tachycardia causes cardiac arrest or shock, immediate cardioversion is indicated (see Chapter 13). Cardioversion should also be undertaken if anti-arrhythmic drugs are ineffective, contraindicated or cause haemodynamic deterioration without restoring normal rhythm. Obviously, cardioversion is inappropriate when ventricular tachycardia occurs in short, self-terminating episodes (Figure 5.9).

Anti-arrhythmic drugs
For prompt restoration of sinus rhythm, drugs are given intravenously. Lignocaine is the first-line drug. Other drugs that are commonly used are mexiletine, disopyramide and flecainide. The last two drugs are markedly negatively inotropic and are best avoided in patients with heart failure or in those known to have extensive myocardial damage. In general, no more than two drugs should be given before considering alternative methods of arrhythmia termination.

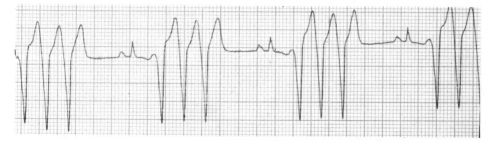

Figure 5.9 Short, self-terminating episodes of ventricular tachycardia

Amiodarone is a very useful second-line drug. It does not have a significant negative inotropic action and is extremely effective. However, it rarely 'works at the end of a needle' and can take up to 24 hours to work. If ventricular tachycardia keeps recurring it is often worth using amiodarone despite its delayed action rather than risking the complications associated with other less effective drugs: even if cardioversion or pacing is required on a few occasions whilst amiodarone is taking effect.

Though verapamil is very effective in controlling supraventricular tachycardias it is, with the exception of fascicular tachycardia, ineffective in ventricular tachycardias. It should not be used as a therapeutic test to ascertain the origin of a tachycardia with broad QRS complexes. Most tachycardias with broad complexes are ventricular in origin; verapamil is unlikely to restore normal rhythm and may cause serious hypotension.

Pacing
Pacing can sometimes be successful in terminating ventricular tachycardia (Figure 5.10). It should be considered when drugs are ineffective, when frequently recurrent tachycardia necessitates multiple cardioversions or when a pacing wire is already in place for treatment of a bradycardia.

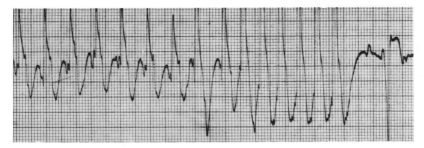

Figure 5.10 Ventricular tachycardia (175/min) terminated by a brief period of overdrive ventricular pacing (225/min)

The usual method is overdrive right ventricular pacing. A burst for a few seconds at a rate 10–30% in excess of that of the tachycardia will often terminate the arrhythmia. However, there is a risk of pacing accelerating the tachycardia or of precipitating ventricular fibrillation; in which case cardioversion will be necessary.

Some ventricular tachycardias are due to a re-entrant mechanism and may be terminated by a pacemaker delivering precisely timed single, double or triple ventricular extrastimuli in the same way that AV re-entrant tachycardia can be controlled. However, there is a risk of extrastimuli initiating a faster arrhythmia. Furthermore, the electrophysiological characteristics and hence response to pacing of a ventricular tachycardia can vary with time, hence long-term pacing is rarely undertaken and is unlikely to be trouble free.

Other electrical devices for tachycardia termination
Transvenous cardioversion – Methods for both temporary and long-term transvenous cardioversion have recently been developed. Much lower energy levels are required for shocks delivered by a transvenous lead as compared with transcutaneous cardioversion. A 'micro-shock' of sufficient energy ($0.5–2.0$ J) will usualy terminate ventricular tachycardia but micro-shocks can be painful and there are problems with implantable devices in distinguishing supraventricular from ventricular tachycardia, i.e. a micro-shock may be discharged inappropriately. As with pacing, there is a risk of actually accelerating the tachycardia.

Implantable defibrillators – These deliver a larger shock: $25–30$ J. Currently, the devices are very expensive and bulky, and use epicardial electrodes which require thoracotomy for attachment. Furthermore, the devices do not always reliably recognize ventricular tachycardia or fibrillation and can provide only a limited number of shocks before having to be replaced. To lose consciousness from ventricular fibrillation and then be defibrillated is not a pleasant experience for a patient. Ideally, the implantable defibrillator should act as a 'backup' device: only to be used if other anti-arrhythmic measures have failed.

In the future, a smaller device which requires only transvenous leads, which can accurately detect a major arrhythmia and deliver the appropriate electrical therapy – extrastimuli, micro-shock or if necessary defibrillation – can be expected.

Prevention of recurrence of ventricular tachycardia

Intravenous drugs
Blood levels of most anti-arrhythmic drugs fall rapidly after a single bolus. After a bolus injection has successfully restored sinus rhythm it is usual to give a continuous infusion of the drug. This makes good sense if ventricular tachycardia is expected to recur within a short period, e.g. after acute myocardial infarction. However, it is pointless to set up an infusion if either the bolus has failed to work or if the tachycardia is known to occur infrequently.

Oral drugs
Unless ventricular tachycardia occurs during acute myocardial infarction or other acute events, recurrence is likely sooner or later and long-term anti-arrhythmic therapy is indicated. Therapy is particularly important if the arrhythmia is associated with significant structural heart disease and/or has caused marked hypotension or shock, since the prognosis without treatment is poor.

Several drugs may be useful: quinidine, mexiletine, disopyramide, flecainide and amiodarone. When ventricular tachycardia has been provoked by exertion beta-blockers are often effective. Disopyramide, flecainide and beta-blockers may precipitate heart failure in patients with extensive myocardial damage. Amiodarone is the most effective of the drugs but often causes unwanted effects. In patients who are at high risk from further arrhythmias it would seem reasonable to use amiodarone and consider alternatives if and when unacceptable side-effects occur.

Occasionally a single drug will not prevent ventricular tachycardia. If the tachycardia is found to be refractory to several drugs given in appropriate dosage it may be necessary to resort to a 'cocktail' of two drugs. The effects of two drugs from different anti-arrhythmic classes are usually combined, e.g. amiodarone plus mexiletine; quinidine plus mexiletine (see Chapter 12).

Sometimes ventricular tachycardia arises during bradycardia. If the heart rate is very low, e.g. less than 50 beats per minute, the rate should be increased by pacing before drugs are given: often pacing alone will prevent ventricular tachycardia.

Pacing together with drugs can be useful in the prevention of ventricular tachycardia when the rate during sinus rhythm is relatively slow, e.g. 50–70 beats per minute,. Pacing at a rate of 80–90 beats per minute will often facilitate control of the arrhythmia.

Surgery

If ventricular tachycardia is refractory to anti-arrhythmic drugs plus or minus pacing, then surgery should be considered. A number of surgical techniques have been investigated, which include the excision or isolation of the arrhythmia focus. However potential candidates for surgery often have impaired myocardial function. Cardio-pulmonary bypass carries a substantial risk when myocardial function is poor particularly since ventriculotomy may worsen function.

Very occasionally, resistant ventricular arrhythmias are an indication for cardiac transplantation.

Assessment of efficacy

Whatever treatment is chosen, it is important to ensure that it is effective in preventing a recurrence of the arrhythmia. It would seem logical to assume that the oral preparation of a drug which when given intravenously had restored normal rhythm, would be effective in preventing a recurrence of arrhythmia. In practice, however, this is often not the case.

If the tachycardia or associated ventricular extrasystoles have been very frequent then monitoring the electrocardiogram at the bedside or using ambulatory electro-cardiography is the best method of assessing the efficacy of anti-arrhythmic therapy. Where control has been difficult to achieve it may be necessary to accept a situation where some ventricular extrasystoles and even short runs of ventricular tachycardia still occur – provided that the rate during tachycardia is significantly slower than before treatment.

If ventricular tachycardia has been an infrequent event then it is unlikely that ECG monitoring will reflect anti-arrhythmic control. Exercise, ECG testing and electro-physiological testing may be helpful.

Ascertaining the cause of ventricular tachycardia

The common causes are listed above. In many cases the cause will be readily apparent from physical examination or electrocardiography. Where the cause is not obvious echocardiography will often be helpful. Occasionally cardiac catheterization may be necessary. Though not clinically indicated, cardiac biopsy may reveal an abnormality in some patients without other evidence of heart disease.

Accelerated idioventricular rhythm

This is defined as ventricular tachycardia with a rate less than 120 beats per minute (Figure 5.11). It is also referred to as idioventricular rhythm and slow ventricular tachycardia. The commonest cause is acute myocardial infarction. Treatment is unnecessary.

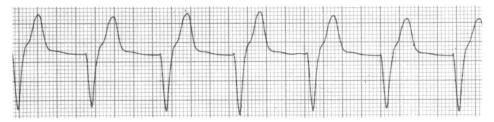

Figure 5.11 Idioventricular tachycardia

Polymorphic tachycardia

Whereas monomorphic ventricular tachycardia consists of a rapid succession of ventricular extrasystoles each with the same configuration, polymorphic tachycardia is characterized by repeated progressive changes in the QRS complex so that the complexes appear to 'twist' about the baseline (Figure 5.12). It is less common than monomorphic ventricular tachycardia but is seen not infreqently after myocardial infarction.

Torsade de pointes tachycardia

This term is used to describe polymorphic ventricular tachycardia associated with prolongation of the QT interval. Its recognition is very important because it may be aggravated by anti-arrhythmic drugs and because correction of the underlying cause should prevent the tachycardia.

The arrhythmia is caused by bradycardia and by drugs or disorders that lead to abnormal ventricular repolarization.

The causes of torsade de pointes tachycardia

- Sick sinus syndrome
- Atrioventricular block
- Anti-arrhythmic drugs
- Congenital prolongation of the QT interval
- Hypokalaemia
- Prenylamine
- Tricyclic antidepressants

Management

Treatment consists of reversal of the cause where possible, and cardiac pacing.

Anti-arrhythmic drugs particularly in large doses or in combination can cause the arrhythmia. The drugs should be withdrawn. Increasing the heart rate to 90–100

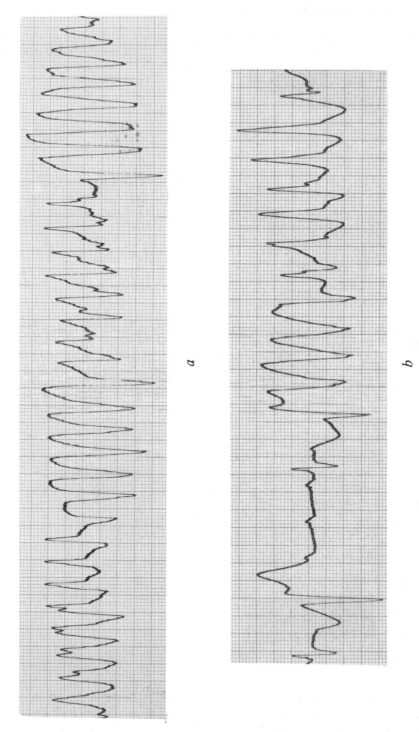

a

b

Figure 5.12 Two examples of torsade de pointes tachcardia: one (*a*) due to prenylamine and the other (*b*) caused by AV block

beats per minute by pacing will often prevent the tachycardia whilst the drug(s) are being excreted or metabolized.

A few patients have a long QT interval even without anti-arrhythmic therapy. In these patients drugs such as quinidine and disopyramide which can markedly prolong QT interval should not be used to avoid the risk of torsade de pointes tachycardia.

There are some reports that intravenous magnesium sulphate may be effective even when serum magnesium is normal.

QT interval

The QT interval is a measure of the duration of ventricular repolarization. It is measured from the onset of the QRS complex to the end of the T wave. Precise measurement is difficult because the timing of these events varies from ECG lead to lead and it is sometimes difficult to define the point at which the T wave ends and U wave starts. Prolongation of the QT interval suggests that either the process of repolarization is uniformly prolonged throughout the myocardium or that the areas of myocardium vary in their rates of repolarization. The latter situation is the one likely to case ventricular arrhythmias.

The QT interval normally shortens with increasing heart rate, partly due to the increase in rate itself and partly due to the increase in sympathetic nervous system activity that is associated with sinus tachycardia. When measuring the QT interval it is necessary to correct the measured interval for heart rate. The following formula is widely used:

$$\text{Corrected QT interval (QTc)} = \frac{\text{measured QT interval}}{\sqrt{\text{cycle length}}}$$

The normal QTc should not exceed 0·42 s.

Congenital prolongation of the QT interval

There are two syndromes in which there are congenital prolongation of the QT interval (Figure 5.13) and tendency to ventricular tachycardia: the Romano–Ward syndrome and the Jervel and Lange–Nielson syndrome. The former is due to a dominant gene;

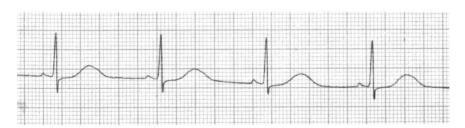

Figure 5.13 QT interval prolongation ($QT_c = 0.57$ s)

the latter is due to a recessive gene and is associated with nerve deafness. Ventricular tachycardia is usually induced by exertion or emotion, i.e. high levels of sympathetic activity and may cause syncope. Sudden death can occur. The disorders are thought to be due to imbalance between left and right sympathetic innervation of the heart. Full beta-blockade is often effective. Occasionally left cervical sympathectomy has been successful.

Main points

- Monomorphic ventricular tachycardia consists of a rapid, regular succession of ventricular extrasystoles each with the same configuration. The QRS duration exceeds 0·12 s.

- The common causes of ventricular tachycardia are myocardial damage from coronary artery disease or from cardiomyopathy.

- The presence of P waves dissociated from ventricular activity or of fusion or capture beats indicates independent atrial activity and confirms a ventricular origin of the tachycardia.

- If the tachycardia causes shock, prompt cardioversion is indicated.

- Lignocaine is the first-line drug for intravenous use. Generally, no more than two drugs should be tried before resorting to amiodarone or non-pharmacological methods of treatment.

- It is important to try to ensure that long-term anti-arrhythmic therapy is effective since ventricular tachycardia is likely to be a recurrent problem and may lead to sudden death.

- Accelerated idioventricular rhythm is ventricular tachycardia at a rate less than 120 beats per minute. Treatment is not required.

- Torsade de pointes tachycardia differs from monomorphic ventricular tachycardia in its ECG appearance, causes and treatment. Anti-arrhythmic therapy may aggravate the arrhythmia and pacing is often effective.

Chapter 6

Tachycardias of supraventricular origin

Several different types of tachycardia originate from the atria or AV junction:

1. Paroxysmal supraventricular (AV re-entrant) tachycardia.
2. Atrial fibrillation.
3. Atrial flutter.
4. Atrial tachycardia.
5. Junctional tachycardia.
6. Sinus tachycardia (see Chapter 1).

It is important to appreciate that within this group of tachycardias there are major differences in mechanism, ECG characteristics and treatment.

The tachycardias have one thing in common: because they arise from above the level of the bundle branches, they usually result in narrow ventricular complexes. This has led some to use 'supraventricular tachycardia' as a blanket term for all the arrhythmias listed above. Others reserve the term for the type of arrhythmia illustrated in Figure 6.1. The mechanism (AV re-entry; as discussed below) which is the usual cause of this arrhythmia and its response to treatment are different from other arrhythmias of supraventricular origin. Its correct title, AV re-entrant tachycardia, has not been widely adopted outside electrophysiological circles.

In this book 'tachycardias of supraventricular origin' will be used to cover the whole group and 'paroxysmal supraventricular tachycardia' will be reserved specifically for a tachycardia due to a re-entry mechanism incorporating the AV junction (Figure 6.1).

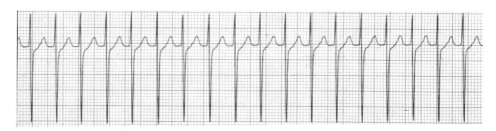

Figure 6.1 Paroxysmal supraventricular tachycardia. It is due to a re-entry mechanism involving the AV junction, hence the term AV re-entrant tachycardia

Paroxysmal supraventricular tachycardia

Mechanism (Figure 6.2)

In most cases the heart is structurally normal, i.e. there is no valve, myocardial or coronary disease. The arrhythmia is due to the repeated circulation of an impulse between atria and ventricles. It can only occur if there are two – rather than the usual one – connections between atria and ventricles. The additional connection either bypasses the AV node (pre-excitation syndromes, see Chapter 7) or is actually within, but functionally separate from, the AV node. The impulse is conducted from atria to ventricles by the normal AV junction and then re-enters the atria via the additional connection.

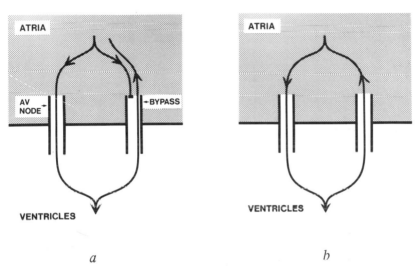

Figure 6.2 Initiation of AV re-entrant tachycardia. An atrial extrasystole arrives at the AV junction while the bypass tract is still refractory to excitation. The extrasystole is therefore only conducted to the ventricles via the AV node. By the time the extrasystole has traversed the AV node and reached the ventricles, the bypass tract has recovered and can conduct the impulse back to the atria (a) thereby initiating the re-entrant mechanism (b)

A variety of terms is used to refer to this arrhythmia. Some reflect its mechanism, e.g. AV nodal re-entrant tachycardia, AV junctional re-entrant tachycardia and reciprocating AV tachycardia; while others are inappropriate, e.g. atrial tachycardia and junctional tachycardia, because these terms are also used to refer to tachycardias due to enhanced automaticity. In this book 'paroxysmal supraventricular tachycardia' will be used instead of these terms.

ECG characteristics

The tachycardia is regular and, unless there is pre-existing bundle branch block or phasic aberrant intraventricular conduction (i.e. bundle branch block caused by tachycardia), the QRS complexes are narrow (see Figures 6.1 and 6.3–6.5). Normal

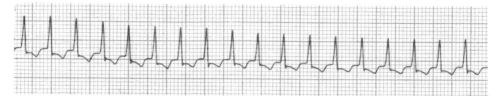

Figure 6.3 Paroxysmal supraventricular tachycardia

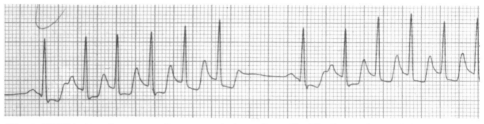

Figure 6.4 Initiation of paroxysmal supraventricular tachycardia. The first and seventh beats are of sinus node origin and are followed by atrial extrasystoles which initiate tachycardia (lead II)

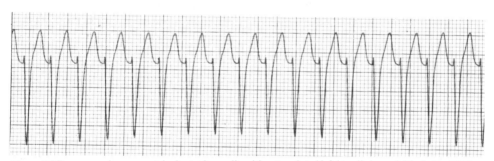

Figure 6.5 Paroxysmal supraventricular tachycardia with rate-related left bundle branch block (lead V1)

P waves will not be seen during this arrhythmia though inverted P waves are sometimes identifiable within the ST segment of the ventricular complex (see Figure 7.8).

The rate during tachycardia can range from 130 to 250 min. In an individual patient the rate is fairly constant but is influenced by the sympathetic nervous system. For example, sympathetic activity and consequently the speed of AV nodal conduction may be increased by assuming a standing position with the result that the tachycardia becomes faster.

Since the circulating impulse re-enters the atria after ventricular activation, *each* QRS complex will be followed by an inverted P wave (see Chapter 7). If the atrial rate is seen to exceed the ventricular rate, whether spontaneously or due to a drug or manoeuvre which slows AV node conduction, then the rhythm is atrial tachycardia or flutter; paroxysmal supraventricular tachycardia is excluded.

The characteristics of paroxysmal supraventricular tachycardia

QRS complexes
- Regular
- Rate 130–250 beats/min
- Usually narrow

P waves
- Inverted, after *each* QRS complex
- Often concealed by superimposed ventricular complex

As with most tachycardias, ST segment and T wave changes can be caused by the tachycardia and persist for some time after its cessation. The ST–T changes are of no diagnostic significance.

In patients with paroxysmal supraventricular tachycardia, the ECG during sinus rhythm is usually normal unless there is pre-excitation (see Chapter 7).

Clinical features

Paroxysmal supraventricular tachycardia is a common disorder. Atacks may start in infancy, childhood or adult life and are often recurrent. The duration and frequency of attacks are variable; they may last for a few minutes or for many hours, and may recur several times per day or be separated by many months. In some patients, attacks are precipitated by exertion. In most, episodes can occur at rest or on exertion and can be precipitated by trivial activities such as bending down.

The main symptom is rapid and often distressing palpitation of abrupt onset. Though the arrhythmia stops suddenly, not all patients are aware of this since tachycardia often follows.

Faintness, syncope, polyuria and chest pain may also occur. Coexistent valvular, myocardial or coronary artery disease may lead to more serious problems. A very prolonged episode of tachycardia, even in a structurally normal heart, may occasionally cause heart failure.

Treatment (see Figure 6.3)
The patient should be reassured that the tachycardia is distressing rather than dangerous and that it is due to an electrical rather than structural cardiac abnormality.

Short episodes of tachycardia without distress do not require treatment.

Summary of treatments for paroxysmal supraventricular tachycardia

Termination
- Vagal stimulation
- Intravenous drugs, e.g. verapamil
- Cardioversion
- Pacing (overdrive, underdrive or programmed stimulation)

Prevention
- Drugs, e.g. sotalol
- Ablation (transvenous or surgical) of AV junction
- Ablation of bypass tract

Vagal stimulation
The first approach should be vagal stimulation. By increasing vagal tone, conduction through the AV node may be slowed and the tachycardia circuit thereby interrupted.

The Valsalva manoeuvre and carotid sinus massage are the best methods. The former is performed by attempting to forcefully expire for 10–15 s whilst the nose and mouth are sealed. Carotid massage is performed by digital pressure over the left or right carotid artery at the level of the upper border of the thyroid cartilage for 5 s. Another widely quoted method of vagal stimulation is eyeball pressure but this is painful and not recommended.

Intravenous drugs
If vagal stimulation does not work, intravenous verapamil (5–10 mg over 30–60 s) will almost certainly terminate the arrhythmia within a couple of minutes (Figure 6.6). Apparent failure of verapamil is usually due to giving too small a dose too slowly. If an adequate dose of verapamil fails to work, the diagnosis should be reconsidered!

Verapamil must not be used if the patient has recently received an oral or intravenous beta-blocking drug (see Chapter 12). Beta-blockers are not as effective as verapamil, and since they preclude use of the latter they should not be employed as first-line treatment. Not infrequently, patients with paroxysmal supraventricular tachycardia are receiving oral beta-blockers. In this case an intravenous beta-blocking drug (e.g. atenolol 5 mg or solatol 20–60 mg) should be tried.

Other drugs such as digoxin, disopyramide and flecainide may also be effective (see Chapter 12). Digoxin does have the advantage of not being negatively inotropic. Disopyramide and flecainide affect conduction in the additional AV connection rather than the AV node.

Electrical methods
If drugs are ineffective or if clinical circumstances necessitate an immediate return to sinus rhythm, cardioversion should be carried out (see Chapter 13).

Various pacing methods can be used to terminate paroxysmal supraventricular tachycardia. The simplest of these is pacing the right atrium at a rate 20–30% faster than the tachycardia (overdrive pacing). On abrupt termination of pacing, sinus rhythm will often return: if unsuccessful, pacing should be repeated several times (Figure 6.7). There is a small risk of precipitating atrial fibrillation which usually will not last for many minutes before sinus rhythm is restored. However, in patients with Wolff–Parkinson–White syndrome atrial fibrillation might lead to a very fast ventricular response (see Chapter 7). Fixed rate right ventricular pacing at 100/min (underdrive pacing) is sometimes effective (Figure 6.7). More sophisticated and efficient pacing methods of tachycardia termination require the use of a programmable pacemaker which allows the introduction of precisely timed atrial or ventricular extrastimuli (Figure 6.7). These pacing methods can be used on a long-term basis by implanting a pacemaker. An intracardiac electrophysiological study is necessary to assess suitability of long-term pacing.

Prophylaxis

A number of drugs may be of prophylactic value, including beta-blockers (especially sotalol), digoxin, verapamil, disopyramide, flecainide and quinidine. Selection of a drug which is both effective and well tolerated is often a process of trial and error. The author usually tries sotalol (160–320 mg daily) first (see Chapter 12). Amiodarone is likely to be effective in cases where other drugs are failed, but should be reserved for refractory cases where the need for tachycardia control outweighs the drug's

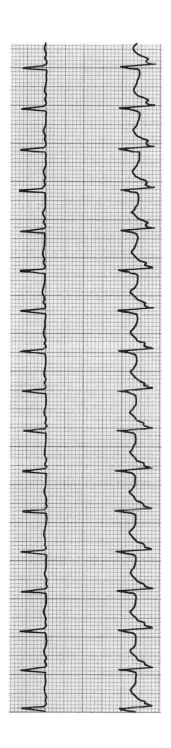

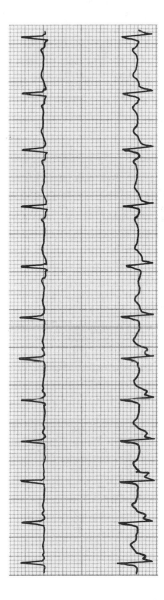

Figure 6.6 Continuous trace: paroxysmal supraventricular tachycardia slowed and then terminated by verapamil (leads I and II recorded simultaneously). There is a P wave immediately following each QRS complex, suggesting that the tachycardia is due to dual AV nodal pathways

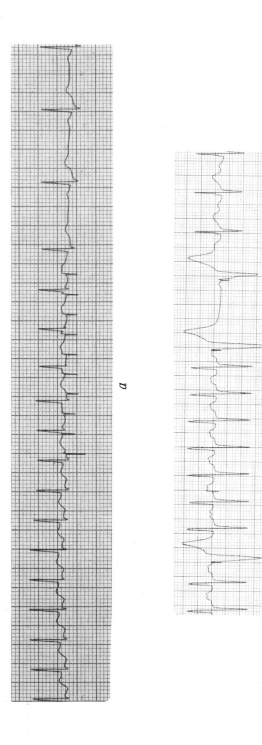

a

b

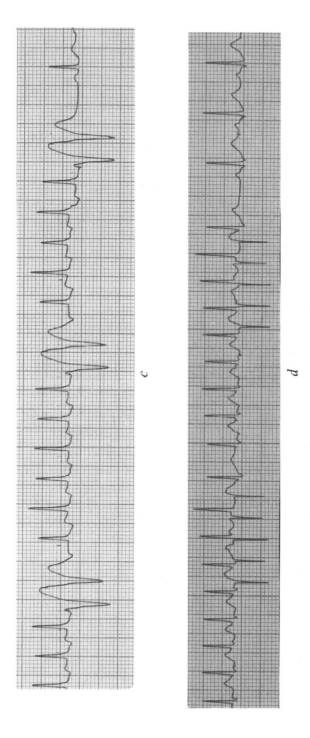

c

d

Figure 6.7 Pacing methods for termination of AV re-entrant tachycardia. (*a*) Rapid atrial pacing. (*b*) Right ventricular underdrive pacing; the second pacing stimulus which captures the ventricles terminates the arrhythmia. (*c*) A scanning implanted pacemaker which introduces a couplet of precisely timed ventricular extrastimuli when tachycardia is detected. After every four cycles, the pacemaker introduces further couplets of extra-stimuli 6 ms earlier in the cardiac cycle until sinus rhythm is restored. (*d*) A scanning, implanted atrial pacemaker

possible unwanted effects. The patient should keep a record of the number and duration of any attacks so that the effect of therapy can be assessed.

In some patients, both drugs and anti-tachycardia pacing are ineffective. An alternative is surgical division of one part of the re-entrant circuit: the AV junction or, if accessible, the additional connection. Recently, non-surgical ablation of AV conduction has been introduced. This is achieved by passing a high-energy (200–400 J) direct current shock to the AV junction via a transvenous pacing lead positioned as close to the bundle of His as possible (Figure 6.8). Methods are being developed to achieve ablation with lower electrical energies and also with alternative sources of energy such as radiofrequency and laser.

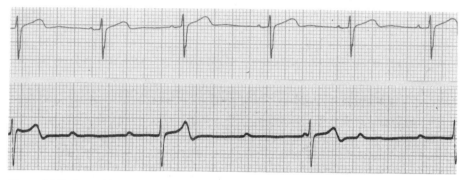

Figure 6.8 Patient with paroxysmal supraventricular tachycardia before (upper trace) and after (lower trace) transvenous AV nodal ablation

Creation of heart block necessitates pacemaker implantation. In most patients who have undergone transvenous ablation, it is necessary to implant a physiological pacemaker which will allow the heart rate to accelerate during exertion: a simple ventricular demand pacemaker will often lead to a markedly restricted exercise tolerance.

A similar technique has been used in some patients for ablation of accessory pathways and foci of origin of atrial and ventricular tachycardias.

A detailed intracardiac electrophysiological study is required to assess the feasibility of ablation and surgery.

Enhanced automaticity

A focus in the atria or AV junction can acquire enhanced automaticity and thereby discharge at a rate in excess of that of the sinus node and take control of the heart rhythm. This is thought to be the mechanism of atrial tachycardia, flutter and fibrillation, and also of junctional tachycardia. (It has been suggested that 'enhanced automaticity' may in fact be due to a re-entrant circuit of only a few cells, but this is not of practical importance.)

Unlike paroxysmal supraventricular tachycardia, which is due to an AV re-entrant circuit, supraventricular arrhythmias due to enhanced automaticity cannot be expected to be terminated by drugs which slow AV nodal conduction. The drugs should, however, reduce the ventricular rate during the arrhythmia. Often with these arrhythmias the purpose of drug therapy is not to achieve a return to sinus rhythm but to control the ventricular response to the ectopic atrial focus.

Atrial fibrillation

In atrial fibrillation the atria discharge at a rate between 350 and 600/min. In the same way that ventricular fibrillation is usually initiated by a ventricular ectopic beat falling on the T wave of the preceding beat, atrial fibrillation is initiated by an atrial ectopic beat falling during the atrial recovery period (Figure 6.9). Fortunately the AV node cannot conduct at a sufficient frequency to allow all atrial impulses to reach the ventricles. After an impulse has been conducted to the ventricles, the AV node will be refractory to excitation by other impulses for a short period. Some impulses only partially penetrate the AV node. They will not, therefore, activate the ventricles but do block or delay succeeding impulses. This process of 'concealed conduction' is responsible for the totally irregular ventricular response characteristic of atrial fibrillation.

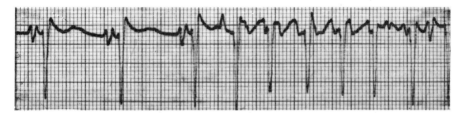

Figure 6.9 Atrial fibrillation is initiated by an atrial ectopic beat superimposed on the ST segment of the third sinus beat

Usually the AV node does not allow a ventricular rate in excess of 200/min, and when AV node conduction is depressed by drugs or disease the ventricular response will be much slower.

ECG characteristics

The rapid and chaotic atrial activity is reflected by 'f' waves which are inscribed at a rate of 350–600/min and are irregular both in rate and size. However, particularly in longstanding cases of atrial fibrillation, f waves may not be seen in all ECG leads. They are usually best seen in lead V1 (Figures 6.10–6.14). Clearly, P waves will be absent.

The hallmark of atrial fibrillation is a totally irregular ventricular response. In the absence of P waves, even if f waves are not seen, a completely irregular ventricular rate is diagnostic of atrial fibrillation. Atrial fibrillation with a rapid ventricular response is often misdiagnosed (Figures 6.15 and 6.16). If the characteristic irregular ventricular rhythm is remembered, this mistake will not be made.

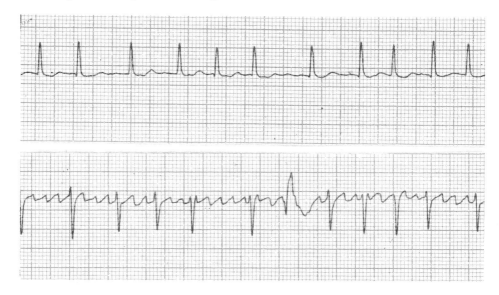

Figure 6.10 Atrial fibrillation (leads 1 and V1). The ventricular rate is irregularly irregular and there are no P waves. 'f' waves are best seen in lead V1 (There is phasic aberrant conduction of the seventh QRS complex in V1.)

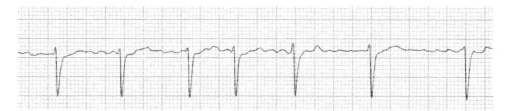

Figure 6.11 Atrial fibrillation (lead V1)

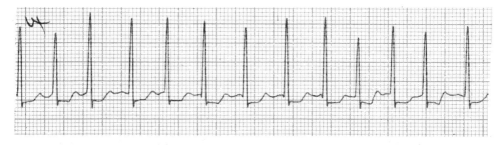

Figure 6.12 Atrial fibrillation. 'f' waves are not seen in this lead but the ventricular rate is totally irregular and there are no P waves

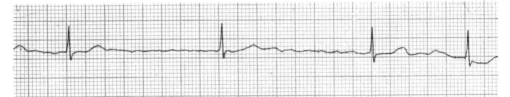

Figure 6.13 Atrial fibrillation with a slow ventricular response

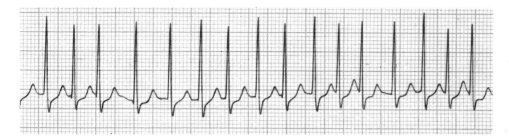

Figure 6.14 Atrial fibrillation with rapid ventricular response

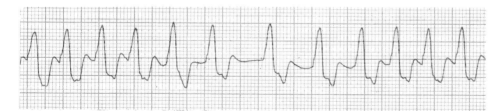

Figure 6.15 Atrial fibrillation with broad ventricular complexes due to pre-existent left bundle branch block (lead V6)

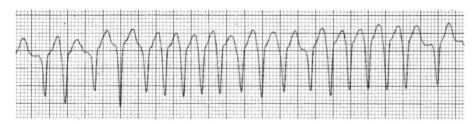

Figure 6.16 Atrial fibrillation in a patient with Wolff–Parkinson–White syndrome. The bundle of Kent facilitates very frequent conduction of atrial impulses to the ventricles and causes broad ventricular complexes due to delta waves

The characteristics of atrial fibrillation

Ventricular activity
- totally irregular ventricular complexes

Atrial activity
- P waves absent
- 'f' waves seen in at least some leads

The only circumstance in which there will be a regular ventricular rhythm during atrial fibrillation is when it is complicated by complete AV block (Figure 6.17).

Sometimes the pattern of atrial activity is so coarse that atrial flutter rather than fibrillation is suspected. In the latter case the atrial rate will usually be greater than 350/min and the ventricular response will be totally irregular (Figure 6.18).

Phasic aberrant intraventricular conduction is often seen during atrial fibrillation. Aberration is the result of unequal recovery periods of the bundle branches. An early supraventricular impulse may reach the ventricles when one bundle branch is still refractory and therefore not capable of conduction whilst the other bundle branch has recovered and will conduct. The resultant ventricular complex will show bundle branch block. The right bundle usually has a longer refractory period than the left and, thus, right bundle branch block is more common. Refractory periods are prolonged with increasing cycle length. Thus aberration is usually seen when a beat having a short cycle length follows one with a long cycle length (Figure 6.19).

Clinical features

Atrial fibrillation is one of the most common arrhythmias. Unlike AV re-entrant tachycardia, atrial fibrillation is often associated with other disease processes, cardiac or non-cardiac, and a cause should be sought.

The main causes are as follows:

The causes of atrial fibrillation

- Rheumatic heart disease
- Myocardial infarction
- Sick sinus syndrome
- Hyperthyroidism
- Alcohol abuse (acute or chronic)
- Myocardial disease:
  Hypertrophic cardiomyopathy
  Dilated cardiomyopathy
  Hypertensive heart disease
  Specific heart muscle diseases
  Myocarditis
- Thoracotomy
- Atrial septal defect
- Constrictive pericarditis
- Pulmonary embolism
- Trauma
- Idiopathic

It should be noted that in a substantial proportion of cases, the arrhythmia is idiopathic and is often referred to as 'lone atrial fibrillation'. In patients in whom the cause is not apparent from clinical examination or from electrocardiography, an echocardiogram should be recorded.

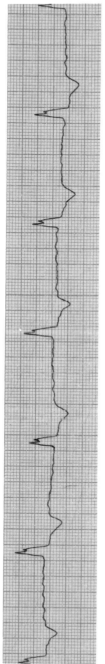

Figure 6.17 Atrial fibrillation with complete AV block. The ventricular rhythm is regular

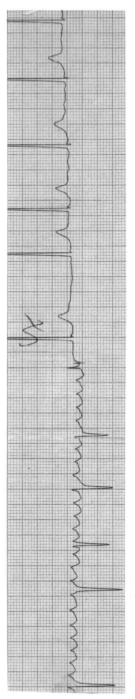

Figure 6.18 Atrial fibrillation. Continuous recording as the lead is changed from V1 to V4. There is a marked difference in baseline activity. The atrial rate is 375/min and the ventricular response is totally irregular

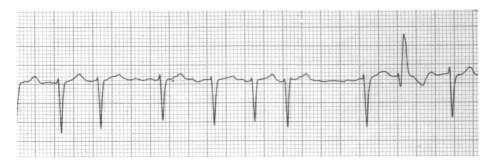

Figure 6.19 Atrial fibrillation (lead V1). The penultimate beat has a short cycle length and follows a beat with a long cycle length. It is conducted with right bundle branch block – phasic aberrant intraventricular conduction

Treatment of persistent atrial fibrillation

Treatment is usually aimed at controlling the ventricular response to atrial fibrillation by the use of a drug or drugs which depress AV nodal conduction. In some patients, the ventricular response is not rapid, even on exercise: AV nodal conduction is probably already impaired and AV nodal blocking drugs are not indicated. Drugs rarely effect a return to sinus rhythm unless atrial fibrillation is of recent onset.

Cardioversion – Cardioversion will often restore normal rhythm but there is a high relapse rate, particularly when there is cardiomegaly, marked left atrial enlargement or when the arrhythmia has been present for a long time. Long-term quinidine or disopyramide do slightly reduce the relapse rate: amiodarone is somewhat more effective but the risk of unwanted effects is not often justified in this situation. When atrial fibrillation has been caused by an acute event, there is a good chance that sinus rhythm will be maintained after cardioversion. Elective cardioversion should be preceded by oral anticoagulation for 2–3 weeks in patients at high risk from systemic embolism (see below). Occasionally in a patient with structural heart disease, atrial fibrillation with a rapid ventricular rate will cause shock and necessitate immediate cardioversion.

Drugs – When a prompt reduction in ventricular rate is required it can be achieved with intravenous verapamil. If verapamil is contraindicated, intravenous digoxin often takes effect quickly. Intravenous amiodarone can also be very useful, particularly when atrial fibrillation is difficult to control after myocardial infarction or cardiac surgery. When there is no urgency, control can usually be achieved with oral digoxin. If in spite of apparently adequate digitalization, control is unsatisfactory, the addition of verapamil 40–80 mg tds or a beta-blocker is usually very effective. Occasionally, the above measures fail in which case one may have to resort to long-term amiodarone or even transvenous ablation of the AV junction.

Treatment of paroxysmal atrial fibrillation

Sotalol is often effective in maintaining sinus rhythm and is usually well tolerated, provided there are no contraindications to beta-blockers. Quinidine and flecainide are sometimes useful. Amiodarone should be considered in patients with troublesome attacks which persist in spite of the above drugs. Verapamil is often prescribed; though it may reduce the ventricular response to atrial fibrillation, it is unlikely to prevent the arrhythmia.

Prevention of systemic embolism

During atrial fibrillation, stasis of blood in the left atrium can occur and lead to thrombus formation and systemic embolism. Patients with rheumatic mitral valve disease are at greatest risk and unless there is a major contraindication should always receive long-term anticoagulation. Indeed, patients with mitral valve disease who are in sinus rhythm should also be anticoagulated – atrial fibrillation is often intermittent before it becomes established.

Patients with atrial fibrillation due to the bradycardia–tachycardia syndrome (see Chapter 10) or acute thyrotoxicosis, and those with a history of systemic embolism are also at significant risk from embolism and anticoagulants should be considered.

Other groups of patients with atrial fibrillation are at much lesser risk from systemic embolism. Embolism is very rare in lone atrial fibrillation. Some have advocated anticoagulation for all cases of atrial fibrillation but this may not be sensible in view of the risks of long-term anticoagulation as compared with the modest risk of embolism. Furthermore, the incidence of atrial fibrillation increases with age, affecting at least 2% of the population over the age of 60 years: the task of anticoagulating a large number of elderly people is daunting.

Atrial flutter

Atrial flutter is less common than atrial fibrillation but the causes are the same. In atrial flutter the atria discharge at a rate between 250 and 350/min. In most cases the atrial rate is very close to 300/min.

Very rarely the AV node conducts all atrial impulses to the ventricles, resulting in a ventricular rate of 300/min. A degree of AV block usually occurs. In patients with a healthy AV node who are not receiving AV nodal-blocking drugs, it is usually 2:1 AV block.

ECG characteristics

The rapid atrial activity is reflected by 'F' waves which are regular. Often there is no isoelectric line between F waves so that the baseline has a 'sawtooth' appearance. Though commonly seen, it is not essential for the diagnosis of atrial flutter. Sometimes, some ECG leads will show the sawtooth appearance whilst others, particularly V1, will show discrete F waves (Figure 6.20).

When there is a high degree of AV block, atrial flutter is easy to diagnose (Figure 6.21). However, when there is a 2:1 AV block, the rapid ventricular response may conceal atrial activity, with the result that the diagnosis of atrial flutter is frequently missed, often being mistaken for sinus tachycardia. The atrial rate in flutter is usually 300/min, and thus during 2:1 AV block the resultant ventricular rate will be 150/min. If this heart rate is found in a patient at rest, it should be assumed to be atrial flutter until proved otherwise. The ECG, particularly lead V1, should be closely inspected for signs of F waves (Figures 6.22–6.24). Often, alternate F waves will be superimposed on ventricular T waves. To confirm that there is an F wave superimposed on the T wave, the interval between the atrial wave preceding the QRS complex and the peak on the T wave must be precisely the same as the interval between the T wave peak

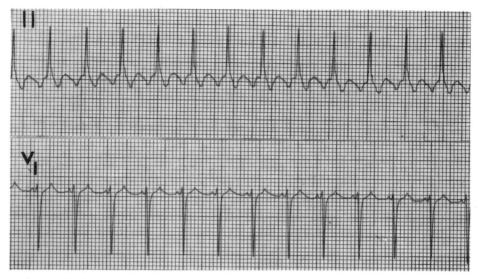

Figure 6.20 Atrial flutter with 2:1 AV block. Lead II shows a classic sawtooth appearance whilst V1 shows discrete atrial waves. In V1 each QRS complex is immediately preceded by an F wave and is followed by an F wave which is superimposed on the T wave

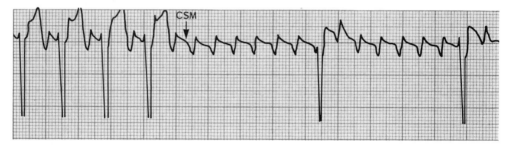

Figure 6.21 Atrial flutter with 2:1 AV block. The degree of AV block increases markedly with carotid sinus massage (CSM)

and the subsequent atrial wave. Carotid sinus massage (see Figure 6.21), or even intravenous verapamil, may be required to increase the degree of AV block temporarily for diagnostic purposes.

The characteristics of atrial flutter

Atrial activity
- 'F' waves at rate of 300 beats per minute
- May have 'sawtooth' appearance in some leads
- Discrete atrial waves may be seen in other leads

Ventricular activity
- Rarely, 1:1 AV conduction resulting in ventricular rate of 300 beats per minute
- Usually, 2:1 or higher degrees of AV bock

When 1:1 AV conduction occurs the ventricular rate will be 300/min. This rate should also be assumed to be due to atrial flutter unless proved otherwise (Figure 6.24).

As with atrial fibrillation, phasic aberrant intraventricular conduction can occur.

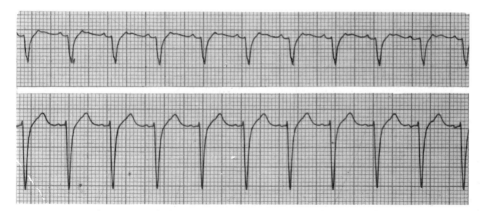

Figure 6.22 Simultaneous recording of leads V1 and V2. Atrial flutter can be readily diagnosed from V1 (alternate F waves are superimposed on the beginning of the ventricular T wave) but V2 looks like sinus tachycardia

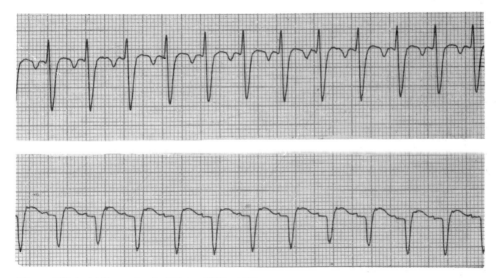

Figure 6.23 Atrial flutter (leads AVF and V1). AVF suggests a sawtooth appearance, V1 shows discrete atrial activity at 300/min: alternate F waves are superimposed on the junction between the QRS complex and T wave

Treatment

Unlike atrial fibrillation, it is often difficult to control the ventricular rate during atrial flutter with AV nodal-blocking drugs. For this reason, if possible, a return to sinus rhythm should be sought.

Atrial flutter can almost always be terminated by cardioversion. Usually, a single low-energy shock is sufficient. Initially, the energy setting should be set at 25 watt-seconds (joules). If unsuccessful, 50 and then 100 J should be tried.

An alternative to cardioversion is rapid right atrial pacing. This has the advantages

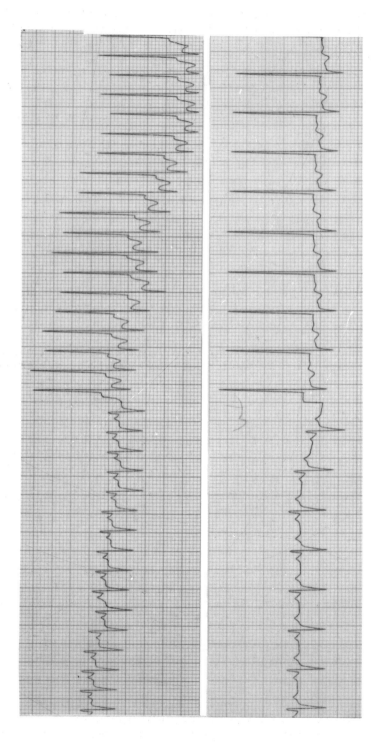

Figure 6.24 Continuous recordings of leads V1 and V4. In the upper trace the ventricular rate is 300/min, suggesting atrial flutter with 1:1 AV conduction. The lower trace shows the effect of carotid sinus massage. The rate is halved and F waves can be seen, in V1, immediately preceding the QRS complex and superimposed on the T wave

that general anaesthesia is not required and that it can be used repeatedly if atrial flutter is a frequently recurrent problem. The necessary pacing rate is usually 10–30% in excess of the atrial rate and should be applied for 10–30 s. On abrupt cessation of pacing, sinus rhythm will return, after a short pause, in approximately one-third of patients. In another third, atrial fibrillation will be precipitated but this often spontaneously reverts to sinus rhythm over the next few hours. In one-third of cases the ryhthm will be unchanged by atrial pacing. It is important to ensure that the pacing stimuli are capturing the atria and this is usually reflected by a change in ventricular rate during pacing.

Atrial flutter may occur in the sick sinus syndrome. When this is suspected, because of the risk of asystole, a temporary pacing electrode should be inserted prior to cardioversion.

In patients with a rapid ventricular rate, intravenous verapamil can be used to increase the degree of AV block temporarily. In about one-fifth of cases verapamil will actually restore sinus rhythm.

In patients with chronic atrial flutter in whom cardioversion has either been unsuccessful or contraindicated, AV nodal blocking drugs are usually required to control the ventricular response unless there is a high degree of AV block. Digoxin should be the initial choice, but it may be necessary to add verapamil. If this combination does not control the ventricular rate, substitution of amiodarone can be very effective: it usually slows both the atrial rate and the ventricular response.

It should be noted that in a few patients with atrial flutter and 2:1 AV block, the increased sympathetic nervous system activity associated with exercise may enhance AV conduction and result in 1:1 conduction and thus a ventricular rate of 300/min. Patients in this situation may experience near-syncope or syncope on exertion.

Atrial tachycardia

The main difference between atrial tachycardia and flutter is that in the former the atrial rate is slower, being between 120 and 250/min. Again, sometimes the AV node can conduct all atrial impulses but often there is a degree of AV block. (With fairly high grades of AV block, because the atrial rate is relatively slow, the rhythm may be misdiagnosed as complete heart block (Figure 6.25) and an inappropriate request made for cardiac pacing.)

ECG characteristics

Because the atrial rate is slower, there is no sawtooth appearance to the baseline. Abnormally shaped P waves are inscribed at a regular rate (Figure 6.25). Usually, the ventricular complexes will be narrow unless there is pre-existent bundle branch block or phasic aberrant intraventricular conduction.

Occasionally atrial tachycardia with 1:1 AV conduction occurs. As in atrial flutter, carotid sinus massage is often helpful in the diagnosis. Again like atrial flutter, atrial activity is often best seen in lead V1.

Causes

Atrial tachycardia with AV block is commonly due to digoxin toxicity (Figure 6.26). The arrhythmia is often referred to as 'paroxysmal atrial tachycardia with block',

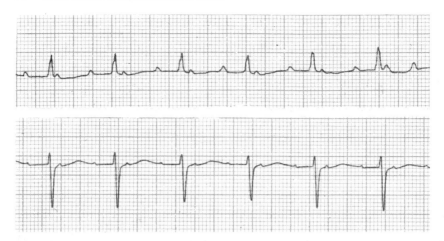

Figure 6.25 Atrial tachycardia with 2:1 AV block (leads AVF and V1). Atrial rate is 175/min

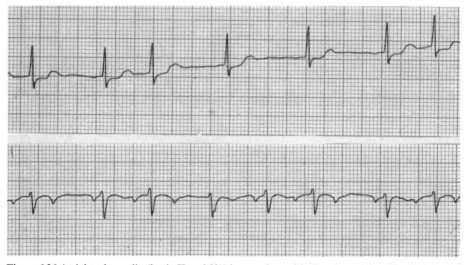

Figure 6.26 Atrial tachycardia (leads II and V1) in a patient with digoxin toxicity. The limb lead suggested atrial fibrillation but V1 clearly shows atrial tachycardia with Mobitz type I AV block

being abbreviated to PATB. The term paroxysmal is inappropriate; particularly in the context of digoxin toxicity, the arrhythmia is usually sustained.

Other causes include cardiomyopathy, chronic ischaemic heart disease, rheumatic heart disease and sick sinus syndrome.

Treatment

If the patient is receiving digoxin, toxicity should be suspected and the drug discontinued. When the patient has not had digoxin, this drug may be used to control the ventricular rate.

If a return to sinus rhythm is required, cardioversion or rapid atrial pacing should be performed.

Junctional tachycardia

Junctional tachycardia is due to enhanced automaticity of the AV junction. It should be distinguished from paroxysmal supraventricular tachycardia which is due to a re-entry mechanism involving the AV node and which is sometimes inappropriately termed AV junctional tachycardia.

ECG characteristics

Usually the QRS complexes are similar to those during sinus rhythm and thus in most cases will be narrow. Occasionally the duration of the QRS complex is slightly longer than it would be during sinus rhythm (Figure 6.27). Usually the junctional focus activates both atria and ventricles. Thus the QRS complex is either preceded by or succeeded by an inverted P wave. Sometimes retrograde atrial activation does not occur and then atrial activity will be independent of the junctional focus.

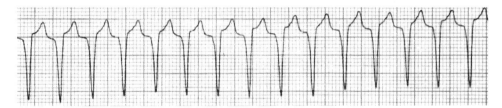

Figure 6.27 Junctional tachycardia (lead V2) in a patient with anterior myocardial infarction

Causes

Junctional tachycardia is commonly caused by digoxin toxicity. Most forms of cardiac disease, especially coronary artery disease, can also cause the arrhythmia.

Treatment

AV nodal blocking drugs may be effective. Otherwise, a drug that decreases automaticity of the focus, e.g. lignocaine or disopyramide, should be used. Where digoxin toxicity is suspected, the drug should be withdrawn.

Main points

- There are several different tachycardias or supraventricular origin. For correct management, it is necessary to determine with which tachycardia one is dealing.

- QRS duration during tachycardia will be normal unless there is pre-existing or rate-related bundle branch block.

- Paroxysmal supraventricular (AV re-entrant) tachycardia requires the presence of a second electrical connection between atria and ventricles in addition to the AV node. Usually structural heart disease is absent. The ventricular rhythm is regular. Atrial activity is usually not seen but if found will be in the form of an inverted P wave after each QRS complex.

- Atrial fibrillation, flutter and tachycardia are due to enhanced automaticity of atrial ectopic foci and are often associated with cardiac or extra-cardiac disease.

- Atrial fibrillation is characterized by a totally irregular ventricular rhythm. Usually AV nodal-blocking drugs are used to control the ventricular response. Though cardioversion often restores sinus rhythm, there is a high relapse rate. Anticoagulation should be considered when the arrhythmia is associated with mitral valve disease, bradycardia–tachycardia syndrome and acute thyrotoxicosis.

- The diagnosis of atrial flutter is based on the finding of atrial activity at a rate of approximately 300/min. Lead V1 is often the best lead for demonstrating atrial flutter: when there is 2:1 AV conduction, alternate F waves will be superimposed on ventricular T waves. Where possible, a return to sinus rhythm should be sought.

- Atrial tachycardia is similar to flutter but the atrial rate is 120–250/min.

Chapter 7

Pre-excitation syndromes

In the normal heart atrial impulses can only be conducted to the ventricles by the AV node. In the pre-excitation syndromes there is an additional connection between atria and ventricles. Unlike the AV node, the accessory connection does not delay conduction between atria and ventricles. Thus atrial impulses will be transmitted more quickly by the accessory connection and will initiate ventricular activation before the atrial impulse has traversed the AV node; hence the term 'pre-excitation'.

The main forms of pre-excitation are the Wolff–Parkinson–White and Lown–Ganong–Levine syndromes.

Wolff–Parkinson–White syndrome

The syndrome is characterized by a short PR interval, a widened QRS complex due to the presence of a delta wave, and a tendency to paroxysmal tachycardia.

Approximately 1·5/1000 of the population have the syndrome.

The Wolff–Parkinson–White syndrome is caused by an accessory connection between atrial and ventricular myocardium. This connection, which consists of ordinary myocardium, is referred to as an accessory AV pathway or bundle of Kent and is congenital in origin. Unlike tracts causing other pre-excitation syndromes, neither end of the connection is to any part of the specialized conducting system. The bundle of Kent may be situated anywhere in the AV groove.

ECG characteristics

Although an atrial impulse will be conducted more quickly by the bundle of Kent than by the normal AV node, once it has reached the ventricles further conduction is relatively slow because the bundle is connected to ordinary myocardium rather than specialized conducting tissues. This slow conduction is reflected by slurring of the ventricular complex, the delta wave (Figure 7.1).

The syndrome is classified into types A and B, depending on the ventricular complex in lead V1. If predominantly positive, it is type A and if negative, type B (Figures 7.2 and 7.3). In type A syndrome the bundle of Kent is likely to be on the left side of the heart and in type B, on the right side. This rule, however is not completely reliable.

During sinus rhythm the atrial impulse will be conducted to the ventricles by both the bundle of Kent and the normal AV node. Because the latter pathway conducts more slowly, initial ventricular activation is solely due to bundle of Kent conduction

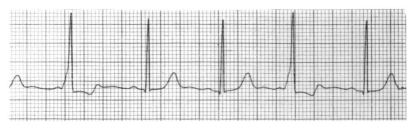

Figure 7.1 Wolff–Parkinson–White syndrome. In this patient, the bundle of Kent conducts intermittently. The second, third and fifth complexes are normal whereas the first and fourth complexes show the characteristic short PR interval and delta wave. By comparing the pre-excited and normal beats, it can be seen how the delta wave both shortens the PR interval and broadens the ventricular complex

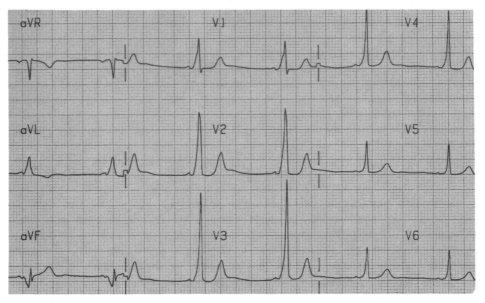

Figure 7.2 Type A Wolff–Parkinson–White syndrome (The negative delta wave in lead AVF could be misinterpreted as a Q wave due to inferior myocardial infarction.)

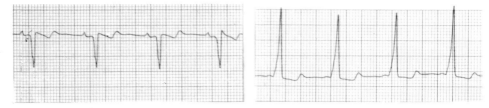

Figure 7.3 Type B Wolff–Parkinson–White syndrome (leads V1 and V6)

which results in ventricular pre-excitation and thus a shortened PR interval. Because the bundle of Kent is not connected to specialized conducting tissue, early ventricular activation will be relatively slow, leading to slurring of the ventricular complex and hence the delta wave. Once the atrial impulse has traversed the AV node, further ventricular activation will proceed normally. During sinus rhythm, therefore, the ventricular complex is a fusion between delta wave and normal QRS complex (Figure 7.1).

Two main arrhythmias can occur in patients with the Wolff–Parkinson–White syndrome – atrial fibrillation and paroxysmal supraventricular tachycardia. The former, which is the less common of the two, is due to enhanced automaticity of an atrial ectopic focus, whereas the latter is caused by AV re-entry.

Atrial fibrillation
In patients without pre-excitation the ventricles are protected from the very rapid atrial activity during atrial fibrillation (350–600 impulses/min) by the AV node. In the Wolff–Parkinson–White syndrome the bundle of Kent provides an additional route of access to the ventricles and is often capable of very frequent conduction. As a result ventricular rates during atrial fibrillation tend to be faster than in patients without pre-excitation and in some patients can be dangerously fast.

Usually, most conducted impulses reach the ventricles via the bundle of Kent and therefore lead to delta waves. The minority of impulses that reach the ventricles via the AV node produce normal QRS complexes. The resultant ECG will, as in all cases of atrial fibrillation, show an irregularly irregular ventricular response. Some ventricular complexes will be normal; most will be delta waves (Figures 7.4 and 7.5).

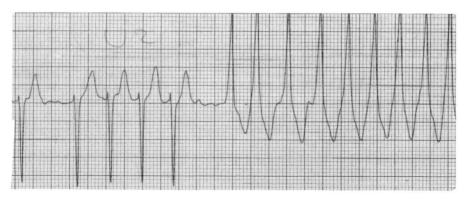

Figure 7.4 Atrial fibrillation (lead V2). The first five complexes are conducted by the AV node and the last nine are conducted by the bundle of Kent and consist therefore of large delta waves

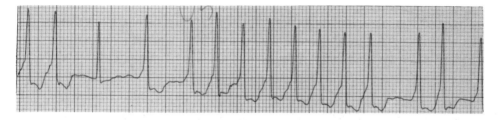

Figure 7.5 Atrial fibrillation (lead V5). Only the third complex is a normally conducted beat, the other complexes are delta waves. There is the characteristic totally irregular ventricular response

A very rapid ventricular response to atrial fibrillation can be dangerous. First, heart failure or shock can result. Secondly, if the ventricles are stimulated at a very fast rate there is a risk of ventricular fibrillation. The risk is confined mainly to those patients where the minimum interval between delta waves during atrial fibrillation is less than 250 ms (Figure 7.6).

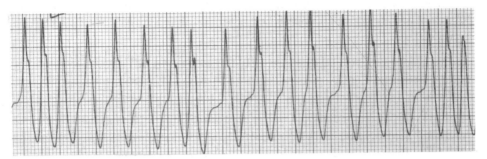

Figure 7.6 Atrial fibrillation with a very rapid ventricular response (leads V1). The minimum interval between delta waves is 180 ms. The totally irregular response excludes a diagnosis of ventricular tachycardia

Paroxysmal supraventricular tachycardia
The AV junction and bundle of Kent differ in the time they take to recover after excitation. Usually, the AV junction recovers first. If an atrial ectopic beat arises during sinus rhythm, when the AV junction has recovered but the bundle of Kent is not yet capable of conduction, the resultant ventricular complex will clearly not have a delta wave and will be narrow. By the time the premature atrial impulse has traversed the AV junction and stimulated the ventricles, the bundle of Kent will have recovered and will be capable of conducting the impulse back to the atria. When the impulse reaches the atria the AV junction will again be capable of conduction and hence the impulse can repeatedly circulate between atria and ventricles. This circus movement is the mechanism causing paroxysmal supraventricular tachycardia in patients with the Wolff–Parkinson–White syndrome. Ventricular ectopic beats may, by a similar process, find one part of the circuit refractory to excitation and initiate a tachycardia.

The ECG during tachycardia will show narrow ventricular complexes (unless phasic aberrant intraventricular conduction occurs) in rapid, regular succession (Figure 7.7).

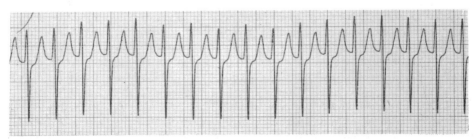

Figure 7.7 Paroxysmal supraventricular tachycardia due to Wolff–Parkinson–White syndrome

Unlike atrial fibrillation, there will be no delta waves and, thus, there will be no clue from the appearance of the ventricular complexes during tachycardia that the patient has Wolff–Parkinson–White syndrome. However, the timing of atrial activity, if it can be identified, during tachycardia may give a clue as to its mechanism. When the tachycardia is due to two pathways within the AV node, i.e. 'dual AV nodal pathway' or 'intranodal' tachycardia (see Chapter 6), an inverted P wave immediately follows or is superimposed on the QRS complex. In contrast, in tachycardias due to the Wolff–Parkinson–White syndrome, the P wave occurs roughly halfway between QRS complexes (Figure 7.8).

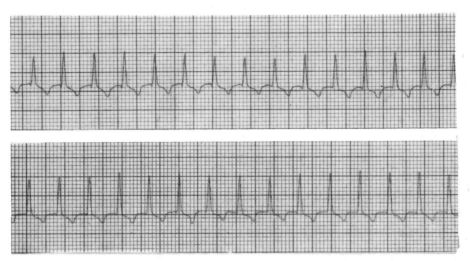

Figure 7.8 Paroxysmal supraventricular tachycardia due to Wolff–Parkinson–White syndrome (leads II and AVF). Inverted P waves can be seen halfway between QRS complexes

The circus movement mechanism of paroxysmal supraventricular tachycardia may be responsible for the initiation of atrial fibrillation: during the circus movement, the impulse circulating between atria and ventricles can stimulate atrial myocardium during its 'vulnerable', recovery phase and thereby precipitate atrial fibrillation (see Chapter 6).

Concealed pre-excitation
Many patients with paroxysmal supraventricular tachycardia who have no evidence of pr-excitation during sinus rhythm have been found to have a 'concealed' bundle of Kent when studied by intracardiac electrophysiological testing (see Chapter 19).

The difference between concealed and ordinary bundles of Kent is that the former can only conduct in one direction. They can transmit impulses from ventricles to atria, the direction necessary to facilitate supraventricular tachycardia, but cannot conduct from atria to ventricles and thus there will be no delta wave or PR interval shortening.

Concealed pre-excitation should be suspected in a patient with a normal ECG during sinus rhythm when, during tachycardia, an inverted P wave is seen halfway between QRS complexes. If inverted in lead I, the bundle of Kent is likely to be left sided (Figure 7.9).

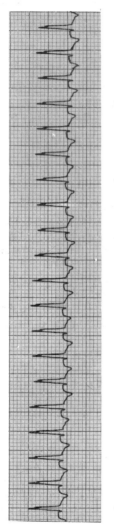

Figure 7.9 Paroxysmal supraventricular tachycardia due to a concealed bundle of Kent (lead I). There is an inverted P wave superimposed on the T wave, halfway between QRS complexes

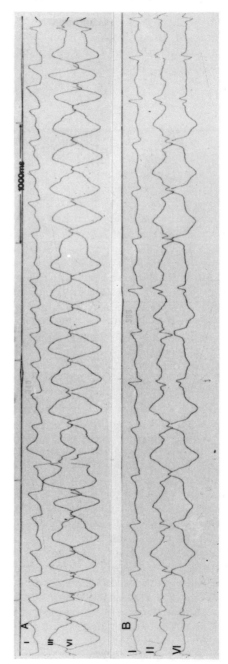

Figure 7.10 Atrial fibrillation in a patient with type A Wolff–Parkinson–White syndrome before (A) and after (B) intravenous disopyramide. ECGs were recorded at 100 mm/s. The minimum interval between delta waves has increased from 180 ms to 400 ms

Treatment

It is often asked, 'What is the treatment for Wolff–Parkinson–White syndrome?' There is no specific 'best' drug or other form of treatment for this syndrome.

Paroxysmal supraventricular tachycardia
Methods for the termination and prevention of paroxysmal supraventricular (i.e. AV re-entrant) tachycardia are discussed in Chapter 6. The methods are appropriate whether or not the patient has evidence of pre-excitation during sinus rhythm.

Atrial fibrillation (Figure 7.10)
During atrial fibrillation, most atrial impulses reach the ventricles via the accessory AV pathway. Thus AV nodal-blocking drugs such as digoxin and verapamil, which are so useful in controlling atrial fibrillation in the absence of pre-excitation, are of little use in the Wolff–Parkinson–White syndrome. Indeed, both digoxin and verapamil can actually increase the frequency of conduction in the bundle of Kent and therefore lead to a faster ventricular rate. For this reason, these drugs should be avoided in those patients who are capable of a rapid ventricular response in case a dangerously fast ventricular rate develops. In patients in whom atrial fibrillation has never occurred, and thus a fast response has not been excluded, digoxin is best avoided.

The simplest method of terminating atrial fibrillation is cardioversion, but this is clearly not appropriate if the arrhythmia is frequently recurrent. If drugs are to be used, they must slow conduction in the bundle of Kent, e.g. intravenous disopyramide, sotalol, amiodarone or flecainide. These drugs will certainly slow the ventricular response to atrial fibrillation and will often effect a return to sinus rhythm.

For prevention of atrial fibrillation, oral sotalol, disopyramide, flecainide, or amiodarone should be considered. In patients with a dangerously fast ventricular response to atrial fibrillation it may be worth initiating atrial fibrillation by rapid atrial pacing once the patient is established on an anti-arrhythmic drug to ensure that the drug will slow the ventricular response to atrial fibrillation.

Surgical division of the bundle of Kent may be necessary when drugs are ineffective or cannot be tolerated, especially if the ventricular response is very fast.

Lown–Ganong–Levine syndrome

The characteristics of the syndrome are a short PR interval, a normal QRS complex and a tendency to paroxysmal tachycardia.

In this pre-excitation syndrome there is an additonal AV connection between atrial myocardium and the bundle of His, which therefore bypasses the AV node. Thus an atrial impulse will reach the ventricles without the normal delay and lead to a very short PR interval. Because the tract is connected to the bundle of His, ventricular activation will be normal and, therefore, there will not be a delta wave (Figure 7.11).

Patients with this syndrome are prone to episodes of paroxysmal supraventricular tachycardia which should be treated normally.

Intracardiac electrophysiological studies have revealed that some patients with the Lown–Ganong–Levine syndrome also have a bundle of Kent.

Not all patients with a short PR interval have an AV nodal bypass tract or are prone by paroxysmal tachycardia.

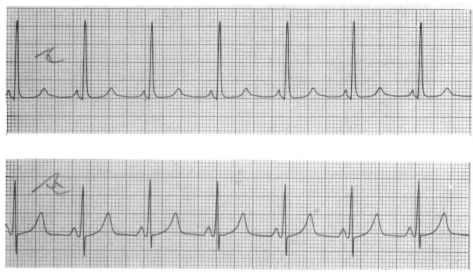

Figure 7.11 Lown–Ganong–Levine syndrome (leads I and II). The PR interval is short but the QRS complex is normal

Main points

◆ The Wolff–Parkinson–White syndrome is characterized by a short PR interval, a widened QRS complex due to presence of a delta wave and a tendency to paroxysmal tachycardia. It is caused by an accessory AV pathway (bundle of Kent), which connects atrial and ventricular myocardium, bypassing the AV junction.

◆ Two main arrhythmias can occur: paroxysmal supraventricular tachycardia (AV re-entrant tachycardia) and atrial fibrillation.

◆ During paroxysmal supraventricular tachycardia, there will be no delta waves and thus no evidence from the ventricular complex that there is pre-excitation. The management of the arrhythmia is the same whether or not there is pre-excitation.

◆ During atrial fibrillation, most ventricular complexes are broad due to the presence of large delta waves. The ventricular rate is often very fast and there is a risk of ventricular fibrillation being initiated when the minimum interval between delta waves during atrial fibrillation is less than 250 ms. If the hallmark of atrial fibrillation (i.e. a totally irregular rhythm) is ignored, ventricular tachycardia may be mistakenly diagnosed.

◆ Since most atrial impulses are conducted to the ventricles via the accessory AV pathway during atrial fibrillation, AV nodal-blocking drugs (digoxin, verapamil) are not helpful. Cardioversion is the simplest method for termination of atrial fibrillation. If drugs are to be used, they must be ones that impair conduction in the accessory pathway (e.g. disopyramide, sotalol, flecainide and amiodarone).

◆ The Lown–Ganong–Levine syndrome is characterized by a short PR interval, normal QRS complex and tendency to paroxysmal tachycardia. It is caused by an accessory AV connection between atrial myocardium and the bundle of His. (Paroxysmal supraventricular tachycardia should be treated in the normal way.) Not all patients with a short PR interval have this syndrome.

Chapter 8

Tachycardias with broad ventricular complexes

Tachycardias of supraventricular origin are sometimes associated with bundle branch block and hence broad ventricular complexes. They may thus mimic ventricular tachycardia. Now that it is widely appreciated that this can occur, the tendency is to misinterpret ventricular tachycardia as supraventricular, rather than the reverse.

Tachycardias with broad ventricular complexes can be due to:

1. Ventricular tachycardia.
2. Supraventricular tachycardia when bundle branch block has already been present during sinus rhythm.
3. Supraventricular tachycardia with rate-related bundle branch block (i.e. phasic aberrant intraventricular conduction).

Useless guidelines

It is often said that whereas ventricular tachycardia leads to major haemodynamic disturbance, supraventricular tachycardia does not. This is incorrect. Sometimes ventricular tachycardia, even due to recent myocardial infarction, causes few or even no symptoms, whereas supraventricular tachycardia, particularly if very fast or in the presence of underlying heart disease, can sometimes cause shock or heart failure.

Another widely quoted rule is that whereas supraventricular tachycardia is regular, ventricular tachycardia is slightly irregular. This rule is unreliable. Ventricular tachycardia is usually regular unless there are capture beats.

Useful guidelines

Clinical circumstances

Myocardial damage caused by coronary artery disease, cardiomyopathy or other disease processes often leads to ventricular tachycardia. On the other hand, myocardial damage is not going to create the additional electrical connection between atria and ventricles which is essential to facilitate the AV re-entrant mechanism which causes paroxysmal supraventricular tachycardia.

Atrial fibrillation (Figures 8.1 and 8.2) is totally irregular and should never get confused with either ventricular tachycardia or paroxysmal supraventricular tachycardia. Though atrial flutter and tachycardia may arise in patients with myocardial

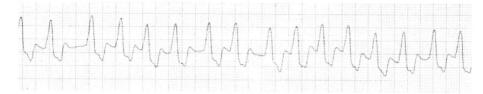

Figure 8.1 Atrial fibrillation with left bundle branch block (lead V6). The ventricular rhythm is totally irregular

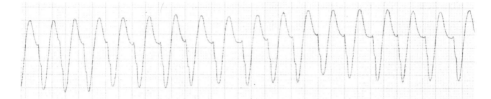

Figure 8.2 Another example of atrial fibrillation with left bundle branch block (lead V3). Though the ventricular rate is more rapid, the rhythm is totally irregular, thus excluding ventricular tachycardia

damage and may be conducted with bundle branch block, there are characteristic features (see Chapter 6) which should lead to their identification.

In practice, a regular broad ventricular complex tachycardia in the presence of myocardial disease is usually due to ventricular tachycardia whereas a supraventricular origin is more likely in a structurally normal heart.

Independent atrial activity

If independent atrial activity (see Chapter 5) can be identified directly (Figure 8.3) or indirectly (Figure 8.4) then supraventricular tachycardia is excluded. (Strictly

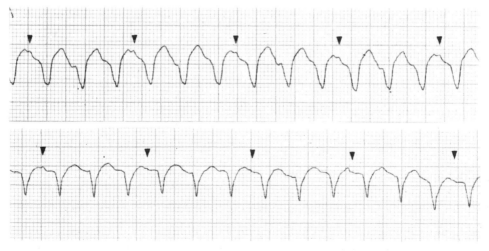

Figure 8.3 Independent atrial activity during ventricular tachycardia (leads AVF and V1). Dissociated atrial activity at intervals of 1·04 s can be identified (arrowheads)

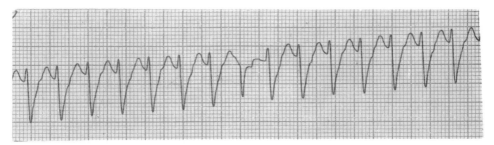

Figure 8.4 Ventricular tachycardia (lead II). The eighth complex is a capture beat

speaking, independent atrial activity can occur in some cases of junctional tachycardia when there is no retrograde conduction to the atria. For practical purposes, however, such a tachycardia is ventricular, since AV nodal-blocking drugs will not be helpful.)

As discussed in Chapter 5, scrutiny of several ECG leads may be necessary to identify evidence of atrial activity (Figure 8.5).

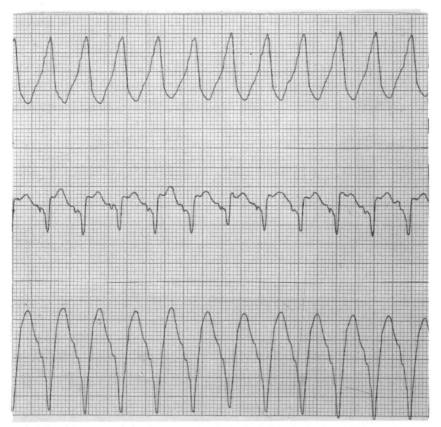

Figure 8.5 Advantage of simultaneous recording of ECG leads (I, II and III). Lead II suggests that there may be a P wave before each QRS complex and thus that the tachycardia is supraventricular in origin rather than ventricular. However, comparison with other leads indicates that the 'P' wave is in fact the initial vector of the ventricular complex

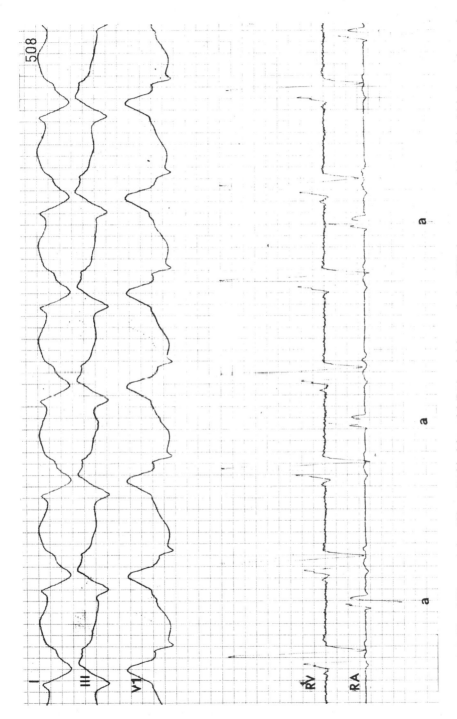

Figure 8.6 Leads I, III and V1 recorded at 100 mm/s with right atrial (RA) and right ventricular (RV) electrograms. Atrial activity (a) is slower than and independent of ventricular activity, indicating ventricular tachycardia

In some patients an atrial electrocardiogram, recorded simultaneously with a surface ECG, is necessary to demonstate independent activity (Figure 8.6). An atrial electrogram can be obtained by passing a transvenous electrode to the right atrium or by using an oesophageal electrode positioned behind the left atrium. An electrically isolated or battery powered ECG recorder should be used.

Carotid sinus massage

Carotid sinus massage can slow AV node conduction and may thus terminate paroxysmal supraventricular tachycardia. If a reduction in ventricular rate occurs during massage but sinus rhythm does not return, it is likely that the patient has atrial flutter or fibrillation; with a higher degree of AV block, flutter and fibrillation waves are more easily identifiable.

Carotid sinus massage is not always effective in paroxysmal supraventricular tachycardia and its failure cannot be taken as evidence for ventricular tachycardia.

Verapamil should not be used as a therapeutic test of the origin of tachycardia; dangerous hypotension may result when the drug is given during ventricular tachycardia.

Configuration of ventricular complex

The broader the ventricular complex the more likely is a ventricular origin. In ventricular tachycardia, the duration of the ventricular complex is often 0·14 s or greater.

Marked axis deviation, left or right, also suggests ventricular tachycardia. Another point towards this arrhythmia is a 'concordant' pattern in the chest leads, i.e. the complexes are either all positive or all negative.

Supraventricular tachycardia may cause bundle branch block, i.e. phasic aberrant intraventricular conduction (Figure 8.7). It is usually the right bundle which is

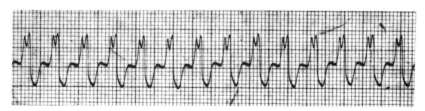

Figure 8.7 Supraventricular tachycardia with left bundle branch block aberration in a case of Wolff–Parkinson–White syndrome (lead V5)

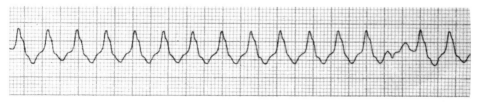

Figure 8.8 Ventricular tachycardia (lead V1). The appearance of the complexes is of right bundle branch block type

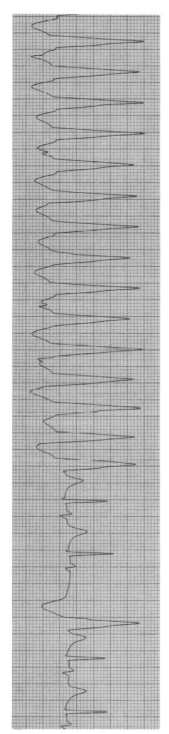

Figure 8.9 The second ventricular ectopic beat initiates ventricular tachycardia. Independent atrial activity can be seen

blocked. Ventricular tachycardia originating from the left ventricle can also result in ventricular complexes with right bundle branch block appearance but the complex in lead V1 is usually biphasic and often has a small Q wave, whereas in aberrant conduction the complex is triphasic and always has an initial positive wave (Figure 8.8).

Retrograde concealed conduction

As discussed in Chapter 3, partial penetration of the AV node by a ventricular ectopic impulse may lead to prolongation of the PR interval during the subsequent sinus beat. Prolongation of the PR interval in the first sinus beat after a tachycardia indicates a ventricular origin.

Ectopic beats

If the configuration of the ventricular complex during tachycardia is similar to that of an ectopic beat recorded during normal rhythm, a common origin is probable. It is relatively easy to ascertain the origin of single ectopic beats, especially if a full ECG is available (Figure 8.9).

Main points

- Though tachycardias of supraventricular origin can be associated with bundle branch block and hence broad ventricular complexes, most wide complex tachycardias are ventricular in origin.

- Pointers towards ventricular tachycardia include the presence of myocardial damage, direct or indirect evidence of independent atrial activity, QRS duration over 0·14 s, a concordant pattern in the chest leads and marked axis deviation.

- Neither minor irregularities during tachycardia or the haemodynamic effect of the arrhythmia are useful in ascertaining its origin.

- When supraventricular tachycardias are associated with aberrant intraventricular conduction, the morphology of the ventricular complexes is usually that of classic left or right bundle branch block.

Chapter 9

Atrioventricular block

The causes of atrioventricular (AV) block are listed below. Idiopathic fibrosis of the AV junction and/or bundle branches is the most common cause.

Causes of AV block

- Idiopathic fibrosis
- Myocardial infarction
- Aortic valve disease
- Congenital isolated lesion
- Congenital heart disease, e.g. corrected transposition
- Cardiac surgery
- Infiltration, e.g. tumour, sarcoidosis, syphilis
- Inflammation, e.g. endocarditis, ankylosing spondylitis, Reiter's syndrome
- Rheumatic fever
- Diphtheria
- Dystrophia myotonica
- Chagas' disease (South America)

AV block is classified as first, second or third degree depending on whether conduction of atrial impulses to the ventricles is delayed, intermittently blocked or completely blocked.

First-degree AV block

Conduction of the atrial impulse to the ventricles is delayed, resulting in prolongation of the PR interval (Figures 9.1–9.3). The PR interval is measured from the onset of the P wave to the onset of the ventricular complex – whether this be a Q or an R wave – and is prolonged if it is greater than 0·21 s.

Usually conduction is delayed in the AV node, but rarely delay occurs within the atria or bundle of His.

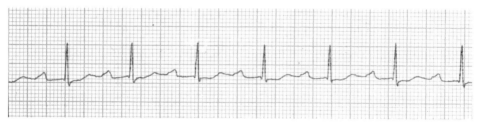

Figure 9.1 First-degree AV block (lead II). PR interval = 0·28 s

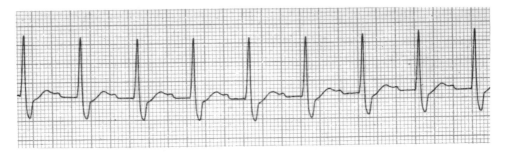

Figure 9.2 First-degree AV block and sinus tachycardia (lead I). PR interval = 0·24 s

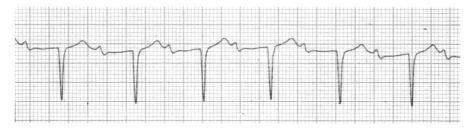

Figure 9.3 First-degree AV block (lead V1). The P wave is superimposed on the terminal portion of the preceding T wave. PR interval = 0·38 s

First-degree AV block does not cause symptoms but may progress to higher degrees of block. In young persons it is usually a benign phenomenon due to high vagal tone.

Second-degree AV block

In second-degree AV block there is intermittent failure of conduction of atrial impulses to the ventricles, leading to dropped beats, i.e. P waves not followed by QRS complexes. Second-degree block is subdivided into Mobitz type I (Wenkebach) and Mobitz type II block.

Mobitz type I or Wenkebach AV block

In this form of second-degree block AV conduction becomes progressively more delayed with each atrial impulse until there is complete block and an atrial impulse fails to be conducted to the ventricles. After the dropped beat, AV conduction recovers and the sequence starts again (Figures 9.4 and 9.5).

AV Wenkebach block is usually due to impaired conduction in the AV node. Like first AV block, it can be benign (particularly when observed during sleep) and is caused by high vagal tone. Recent evidence suggests that Wenkebach block which cannot be attributed to high vagal tone has a similar prognosis to Mobitz II block (see Chapter 16).

The increments in AV-nodal conduction delay are usually greatest at the start of the Wenkebach sequence. This leads to the somewhat paradoxical finding that, as

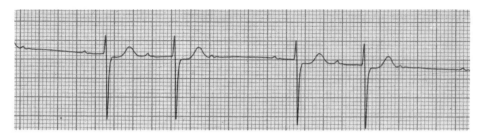

Figure 9.4 AV Wenkebach block. Unlike many textbooks examples, but as often occurs in practice, the trace does not start with the shortest PR interval

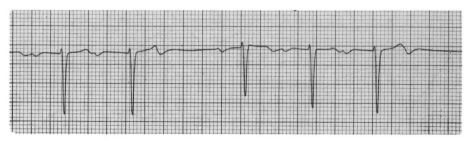

Figure 9.5 AV Wenkebach block. The non-conducted P wave is superimposed on the preceding T wave

the sequence approaches the dropped beat, the QRS complexes actually become closer together.

Mobitz type II AV block

In Mobitz type II block there is intermittent failure of conduction of atrial impulses to the ventricles without antedecent progressive lengthening of the PR interval, and thus the PR interval of conducted beats is constant (Figure 9.6).

In contrast to first-degree and Wenkebach AV block, Mobitz type II block is usually due to impaired conduction in the bundle of His or bundle branches (i.e. infranodal). Thus, because there is bundle branch disease, the QRS complexes are usually broad. Block below the AV node is more likely to be associated with Stokes–Adams attacks, slow ventricular rates and sudden death.

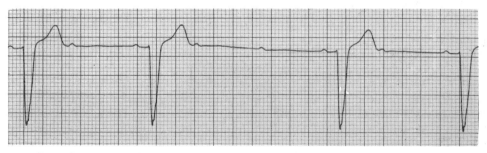

Figure 9.6 Mobitz type II AV block. In this example the ratio between conducted and non-conducted atrial impulses varies

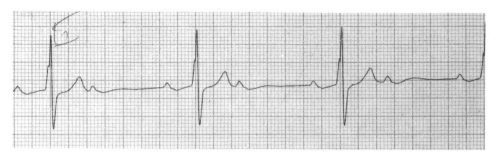

Figure 9.7 Mobitz type II AV block with 2:1 AV conduction

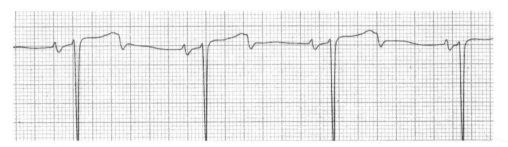

Figure 9.8 2:1 AV block with narrow QRS complexes (lead V1). The non-conducted atrial beats are superimposed on preceding T-waves

The ratio of conducted to non-conducted atrial impulses varies. Commonly 2:1 AV conduction occurs (Figure 9.7). A similar pattern may be caused by an extreme form of Wenkebach block so that it is difficult to make prognostic inferences from 2:1 AV block (Figure 9.8).

Usually, during Mobitz type II block, the atrial rate is regular. Sometimes, however, the P–P interval encompassing a ventricular complex is shorter than a P–P interval which does not. This is known as ventriculophasic sinus arrhythmia.

Third-degree AV block

Third-degree or complete AV block occurs when there is total interruption of the transmission of atrial impulses to the ventricles. Third-degree block may be due to interrupted conduction at either AV nodal or infranodal level. When the block is within the AV node, subsidiary pacemakers arise within the bundle of His and, unless there is additional bundle branch block, will lead to narrow QRS complexes (Figure 9.9). Often, pacemakers within the bundle of His discharge reliably at a fairly rapid rate.

In contrast, in intranodal block subsidiary pacemakers usually arise in the left or right bundle branches. These pacemakers will produce broad QRS complexes and slower ventricular rates (Figures 9.10 and 9.13). Pacemaker activity is less reliable and thus Stokes–Adams attacks are more likely.

Complete AV block can complicate atrial fibrillation and flutter (Figures 9.11 and 9.12).

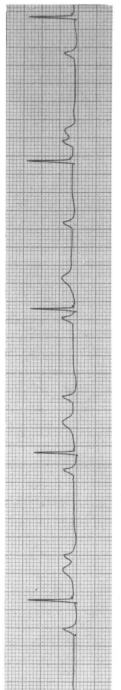

Figure 9.9 Complete AV block with narrow QRS complexes

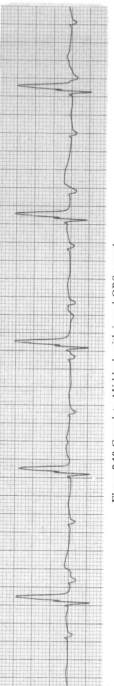

Figure 9.10 Complete AV block with broad QRS complexes

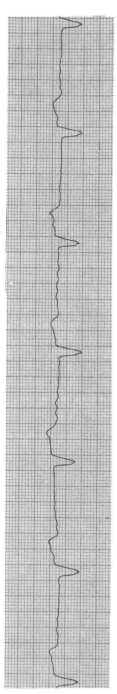

Figure 9.11 Complete AV block with atrial fibrillation

Occasionally, heart block only occurs during exercise and can be the cause of exertional syncope or weakness.

Supernormal conduction
Occasionally, even during third-degree AV block, atrial impulses may be conducted to the ventricles. There is a short period immediately after recovery from excitation when AV conduction may transiently improve. This period usually coincides with inscription of the latter portion of the T wave (Figure 9.13). As a result, atrial impulses falling on this part of the T wave will be followed by a premature QRS complex.

AV dissociation

During third-degree AV block, atrial activity is faster than and dissociated from ventricular activity. Dissociation between atrial and ventricular activity also occurs when, often during sinus bradycardia, an escape rhythm faster than the sinus rate arises in the AV junction or ventricles (Figure 9.14). The term 'AV dissociation' should be reserved for this latter situation, in which the ventricular rate is *greater* than the atrial rate. If AV dissociation is not distinguished from complete AV block, inappropriate action can result. For example, AV dissociation often occurs in acute myocardial infarction and, if not recognized as such, a pacemaker may be unnecessarily inserted.

During AV dissociation, the timing of some P waves may be such that they can be transmitted by the AV junction and capture the ventricles before the next discharge from the escape junctional or ventricular focus and therefore lead to premature ventricular activation. This is known as 'AV dissociation with capture beats'.

Bilateral bundle branch disease

Infranodal AV block may be due to a lesion in the bundle of His but is more often caused by disease in both left and right bundle branches.

Although the anatomical situation may be more complex, functionally the bundle of His can be considered to divide into three: the right bundle branch and the anterior and posterior fascicles of the left bundle branch (see Chapter 4).

If conduction is blocked in only two of the three fascicles (bifascicular block), the functioning fascicle will conduct atrial impulses to the ventricles and maintain sinus rhythm. Block in the third fascicle will lead to complete AV block.

Bifascicular block

The most common pattern of bifascicular block is right bundle branch plus left anterior fascicular block (Figure 9.15). The posterior fascicle of the left bundle branch is a stouter structure and has a better blood supply than the anterior fascicle and is therefore less vulnerable. As a resut, right bundle branch plus left posterior fascicular block is a less common occurrence (Figure 9.16).

Block in anterior and posterior fascicles of the left bundle branch causes complete left bundle branch block. The combination of left bundle branch block and left axis deviation may indicate more disease of conduction tissues than left bundle branch block with a normal frontal axis (Figure 9.17).

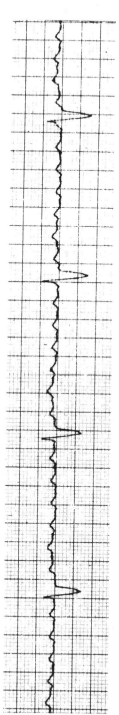

Figure 9.12 Complete AV block with atrial flutter

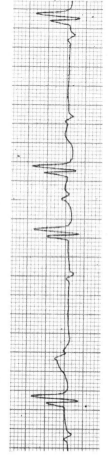

Figure 9.13 Complete AV block. There is supernormal conduction of the atrial impulse that falls on the T wave on the second ventricular complex (lead V1)

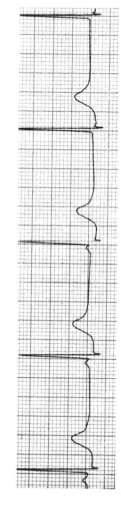

Figure 9.14 AV dissociation. Atrial and ventricular rates are 49 and 51/min, respectively. The fourth and fifth P waves are concealed by superimposed QRS complexes

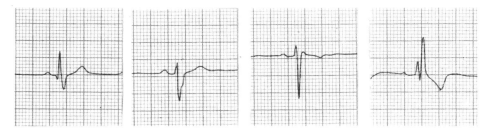

Figure 9.15 Left anterior fascicular and right bundle branch block (leads I, II, III and V1)

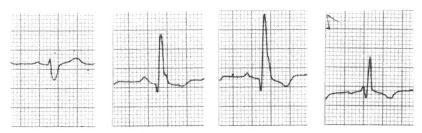

Figure 9.16 Left posterior fascicular and right bundle branch block (leads I, II, III and V1)

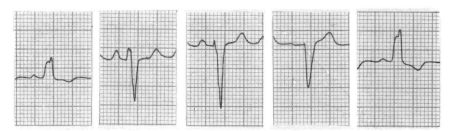

Figure 9.17 Left axis deviation and left bundle branch block (leads I, II, IIII, V1 and V6)

PR interval prolongation is usually due to impaired AV node conduction, but in the context of bifascicular block it is more likely to reflect abnormal conduction in the functioning fascicle.

Trifascicular block

Interrupted conduction in all three fascicles results in complete AV block. In many patients one of the three fascicles is capable of intermittent conduction so that, for part of the time, there will be sinus rhythm with evidence of bifascicular block.

The risk of bifascicular block progressing to trifascicular block is fairly low. In patients with right bundle and left anterior fascicular block, this is in the order of a few per cent per year. The risk is increased when there is right bundle and left posterior fascicular block and when there is alternating complete right and left bundle branch block. There is little evidence to suggest that prophylactic implantation of a permanent pacemaker in asymptomatic patients with bifascicular block improves prognosis. The major determinants of prognosis are the states of the myocardium and coronary arteries.

Clinical features of AV block

First-degree and Mobitz type I second-degree AV block do not cause symptoms but may progress to higher grades of block.

In Mobitz type II and complete AV block, a low ventricular rate may cause tiredness, dyspnoea and heart failure. In some patients the ventricular pacemaker may at times discharge very slowly or actually stop, leading to syncope or, if ventricular activity does not quickly return, sudden death. Ventricular fibrillation and tachycardia arise in some patients as a consequence of the low ventricular rate and may also lead to syncope or sudden death.

Stokes–Adams attacks

Syncope due to transient asystole or ventricular fibrillation – a Stokes–Adams attack – has characteristic features. These features are of great diagnostic importance because, on the one hand, abnormalities of AV conduction (and sinus node function) may be intermittent, routine electrocardiography being normal, and on the other hand, in patients with evidence of disease of the specialized conducting tissues, syncope may be due to unrelated causes such as epilepsy.

In a Stokes–Adams attack, loss of consciousness is abrupt. There is virtually no warning, though the patient will sometimes feel that he is going to faint, just before he loses consciousness. The patient collapses, lying motionless, pale and pulseless. He looks as though he is dead. In a prolonged attack twitching may develop and progress to a fit. Usually, within a minute or two, consciousness returns, and as cardiac action resumes there is a vivid flush to the skin. Incontinence does occur occasionally but is not a regular feature as it is in epilepsy. Unlike epilepsy, recovery is quick and confusion and headache after the attack are unusual.

In some patients the rhythm disturbance does not last long enough to cause syncope but the patient feels as though he is going to faint (near-syncope) and then recovers. He may complain of 'dizziness' but will not experience true vertigo.

Congenital heart block

This is a relatively benign disorder. AV conduction is interrupted at the AV nodal level. Consequently, the subsidiary ventricular pacemaker is situated in the proximal part of the bundle of His (producing narrow QRS complexes) and discharges reliably at a relatively fast rate (40–80/min) which may accelerate on exercise. Usually there are no symptoms and exercise tolerance is good.

However, syncope and sudden death do occur in a minority of patients (see Chapter 16).

Acquired heart block

Heart block complicating myocardial infarction is discussed in Chapter 11.

As discussed above, the commonest cause of heart block is idiopathic fibrosis of the AV junction or bundle branches. This mainly affects the elderly but – as with the other causes of AV block – can affect the young and middle aged as well.

The bradycardia associated with Mobitz type II and third-degree AV block may reduce cardiac output and lead to symptoms such as shortness of breath, tiredness and heart failure. Stokes–Adams attacks will sooner or later occur in about two-thirds of patients with these higher grades of AV block.

Treatment

Artificial cardiac pacing has greatly improved the symptoms and prognosis. The indications are discussed in Chapters 15 and 16.

Main points

♦ AV block is classified as first, second or third degree depending on whether conduction of atrial impulses to the ventricles is delayed, intermittently blocked or completely blocked.

♦ Second-degree AV block is subdivided into Mobitz I (Wenkebach) and Mobitz II types. In the former, there is progressive lengthening of the PR interval prior to non-conduction of an atrial impulse, whereas the PR interval of conducted atrial impulses is constant in Mobitz II.

♦ During AV dissociation (in contrast to complete AV block), the atrial rate is slower than the ventricular rate.

♦ First-degree block, Wenkebach block and third-degree block with narrow QRS complexes are usually due to disease within the AV node, whereas Mobitz II and complete block with broad QRS complexes are likely to be due to infranodal block.

♦ Bifascicular block may deteriorate intermittently or permanently to complete (trifascicular) AV block.

♦ Stokes–Adams attacks are characterized by abrupt loss of consciousness which lasts for a few minutes only, following which recovery is usually rapid. Patients with conduction tissue disease often experience 'near-syncope' as well as episodes of complete loss of consciousness.

Chapter 10

Sick sinus syndrome

The sick sinus syndrome, also referred to as sino-atrial disease, is caused by impairment of either sinus node activity or of conduction of impulses from the sinus node to the atria. The result is sinus bradycardia, sino-atrial block or sinus arrest.

In some patients tachycardias of supraventricular origin may also occur. The term 'bradycardia–tachycardia' (often abbreviated to 'brady–tachy') syndrome is applied to these patients.

Sick sinus syndrome is a common cause of syncope, dizzy attacks and palpitation. Though found most frequently in the elderly, it can occur at any age.

Causes

The cause is usually idiopathic fibrosis of the sinus node. Sick sinus syndrome can be due to acute myocardial infarction, chronic ischaemic heart disease, cardiomyopathy, myocarditis, digoxin or quinidine toxicity, or cardiac surgery, especially atrial septal defect repair. Sometimes, anti-arrhythmic drugs may precipitate an otherwise latent disorder.

ECG characteristics

Any one of the following abnormal rhythms can occur. They are often intermittent, normal sinus rhythm being present for most of the time.

Sinus bradycardia

Sinus bradycardia is a common finding in the sick sinus syndrome. The rate may fall as low as 30 beats/min.

Sinus arrest

Sinus arrest is due to failure of the sinus node to activate the atria because of cessation of sinus node activity. The result is absence of normal P waves (Figures 10.1 and 10.2).

Physiological studies have shown that in the absence of sinus node activity, subsidiary pacemakers in the atria, AV junction or ventricles should give rise to an escape rhythm. In the sick sinus syndrome, however, the subsidiary pacemakers are

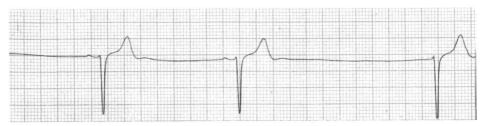

Figure 10.1 Sinus bradycardia and then sinus arrest leading to a junctional escape beat

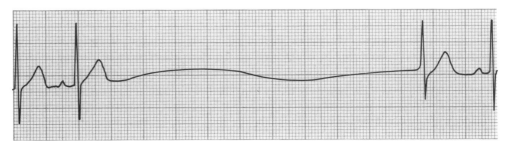

Figure 10.2 Sinus arrest leading to a prolonged period of ventricular standstill, eventually terminated by a junctional escape beat

often far from reliable and sinus arrest may therefore lead to cardiac standstill. Thus, although sinus arrest is attributed to disordered sinus node function, where asystole occurs, there is also abnormal function of the more distal specialized conducting system (Figure 10.2).

Sinus bradycardia and sino-atrial block during sleep are physiological and should not be taken as evidence for the sick sinus syndrome. Furthermore, pauses in sinus node activity of up to 2·0 s due to high vagal tone may be found in fit, young people.

Sino-atrial block

Sino-atrial block occurs when sinus node impulses fail to traverse the junction between the node and surrounding atrial myocardium. Like atrioventricular block, sino-atrial block can be classified into first, second or third degree. However, only second-degree sino-atrial block can be confidently diagnosed from the ECG. Third-degree or complete sino-atrial block is indistinguishable from sinus arrest.

In second-degree sino-atrial block, there are intermittently dropped P waves, resulting in intervals between P waves which are multiples of (often twice) the cycle length during sinus rhythm (Figure 10.3).

Escape beats and rhythms

When sinus bradycardia or arrest occurs, subsidiary pacemakers may give rise to an escape beat or rhythm (see Figures 10.1, 10.2 and 10.4). Presence of a junctional or idioventricular rhythm suggests abnormal sinus node function.

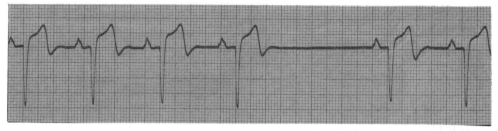

Figure 10.3 Second-degree sino-atrial block. Both the P wave and QRS complex are dropped for one cycle

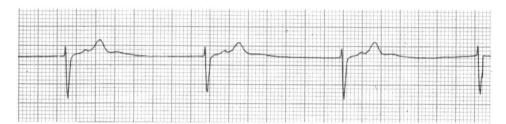

Figure 10.4 Junctional escape rhythm secondary to sinus arrest. The functional focus activates the atria retrogradely leading to P waves superimposed on the ST segments

Atrial ectopic beats

These are often found in the sick sinus syndrome (Figure 10.5). Characteristically they are followed by long pauses because sinus node automaticity is depressed by the ectopic beat (Figure 10.6).

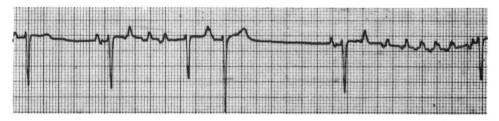

Figure 10.5 Atrial ectopic beats after the second, third and fifth QRS complexes. On two occasions brief episodes of atrial flutter are initiated

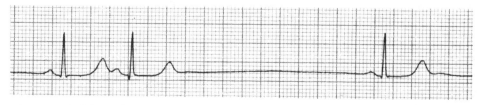

Figure 10.6 Atrial ectopic beat leads to a depression of sinus node automaticity

Bradycardia–tachycardia syndrome

Several tachycardias of supraventricular origin may occur in patients with the sick sinus syndrome. Paroxysmal atrial fibrillation and flutter are the most common (Figures 10.5 and 10.7). Atrial and junctional tachycardia also occur. However, paroxysmal supraventricular (i.e. AV re-entrant) tachycardia (see Chapter 6) is not associated with this syndrome.

Sinus node automaticity is often depressed by these tachycardias so that termination of the tachycardia is followed by a period of sinus bradycardia or arrest. Conversely, tachycardias often arise as an escape rhythm following bradycardia. Thus tachycardia often alternates with bradycardia.

AV junction disease

Abnormal AV conduction is not infrequently found in patients with sick sinus syndrome (Figure 10.8). In patients with sick sinus syndrome who develop atrial fibrillation there is often a slow ventricular response in the absence of digoxin or other AV nodal-blocking drugs suggesting coexistent impaired AV nodal function (Figure 10.9).

Clinical features

Sinus arrest without an adequate escape rhythm may cause syncope or dizzy attacks, depending on its duration. Tachycardias often produce palpitation, and resultant sinus node depression may lead to syncope or near-syncope after palpitation.

The frequency of rhythm disturbance is very variable. Some patients will experience symptoms many times per day whereas in others symptoms may be separated by intervals of several months.

In the absence of mitral valve disease, atrial tachyarrhythmias rarely cause systemic embolism. The bradycardia–tachycardia syndrome is an exception to this rule. Incidences of up to 15% have been reported.

Diagnosis

Sick sinus syndrome should be suspected when there are symptoms of syncope, near-syncope or palpitation in the presence of sinus bradycardia or an escape rhythm. Prolonged sinus arrest or sino-atrial block confirms the diagnosis.

Sometimes diagnostic information can be obtained from the standard ECG but often 24-hour ambulatory ECG recordings will be necessary. Both sinus bradycardia and tachycardia can be physiological. Not infrequently, an erroneous diagnosis of bradycardia–tachycardia syndrome is made from a 24 hour tape recording which merely shows sinus bradycardia during sleep and sinus tachycardia during exertion!

Occasionally, when symptoms and rhythm disturbances are infrequent, intracardiac electrophysiological testing may be helpful (see Chapter 19).

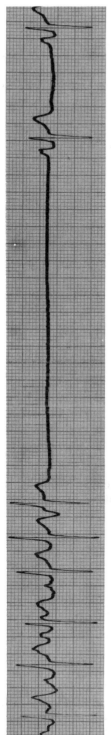

Figure 10.7 Termination of atrial fibrillation followed by sinus arrest

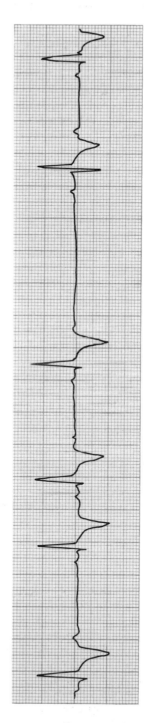

Figure 10.8 Intermittent Mobitz type II AV block and periods of sinus arrest

Treatment

Sinus bradycardia or arrest

With the exception of sinus node dysfunction in acute myocardial infarction, where atropine may be helpful, drugs are ineffective in preventing sinus bradycardia or arrest and may precipitate tachyarrhythmias. Cardiac pacing is necessary to control symptoms.

For two reasons atrial pacing is preferable to ventricular pacing. First, atrial pacing maintains the normal sequence of cardiac number activation. With ventricular pacing the loss of atrial contribution to ventricular filling may result in a reduction of cardiac output of up to 30% (see Chapter 16). The second advantage to atrial pacing is that regular atrial systole reduces the risk of systemic emboli. In patients with both sinus node and AV junction disease, A–V sequential pacing can be carried out (see Chapter 16).

Bradycardia–tachycardia syndrome

Anti-arrhythmic drugs, especially beta-blockers and disopyramide, often worsen sinus node function and thus increase the risk of syncope. It is usually necessary to implant a pacemaker if anti-arrhythmic drugs are required to control tachycardias, particularly if sino-atrial block or arrest has occurred.

Tachycardias often arise as an escape rhythm during bradycardia. Atrial pacing may prevent initiation of tachyarrhythmias by ensuring regular atrial activity.

Cardioversion may cause asystole and should be preceded by insertion of a temporary pacemaker.

Systemic embolism

Because of the risk of systemic embolism, some would recommend long-term anticoagulation for patients in whom atrial tachyarrhythmias cannot be prevented. Anticoagulants are certainly indicated when there is a history of embolism.

Carotid sinus syndrome

This term refers to a group of patients who suffer from near-syncope or syncope without electrocardiographic evidence of sinus node or AV junctional disease in whom unilateral carotid sinus massage (for 5 s) causes sinus arrest or complete AV block for 3 s or more (Figure 10.10). In some of these patients baroreceptor stimulation also causes marked hypotension.

It should be noted that some subjects, particularly among the elderly, who are entirely asymptomatic, may develop a marked bradycardia on carotid massage. In symptomatic patients, atrial or AV sequential pacing is required.

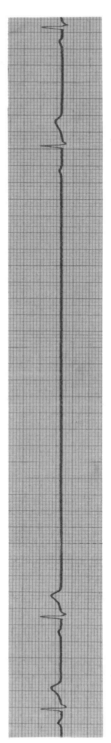

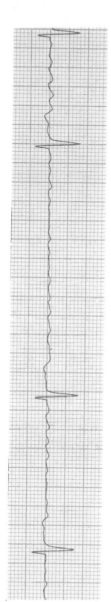

Figure 10.9 Atrial fibrillation with slow ventricular response in a patient who also had periods of sinus bradycardia and arrest

Figure 10.10 Carotid sinus syndrome. Carotid massage led to asystole for 5 s

Main points

- The sick sinus syndrome is due to impaired sinus node function and/or sino-atrial conduction and may cause sinus bradycardia, sino-atrial block or sinus arrest.

- A substantial pause in sinus node activity without an adequate junctional or ventricular escape rhythm will cause near-syncope or syncope.

- The bradycardia–tachycardia syndrome consists of the occurrence of both sinus node dysfunction and episodes of atrial fibrillation, flutter or tachycardia. Often, bradycardia will alternate with tachycardia. AV re-entrant tachycardia does not occur as part of this syndrome.

- Artificial pacing is required for control of symptoms due to the sick sinus syndrome and to prevent profound bradycardia if anti-arrhythmic drugs are to be prescribed for the bradycardia–tachycardia syndrome.

Chapter 11

Arrhythmias in myocardial infarction

A wide variety of arrhythmias may be caused by acute myocardial infarction (Table 11.1). Some necessitate immediate treatment whereas no treatment is required for others. Arrhythmias are most frequent in the early hours after infarction.

Table 11.1 Incidence of arrhythmias (%) observed in a series of patients within 4 hours of myocardial infarction

Ventricular fibrillation	16
Ventricular tachycardia	4
Ventricular ectopic beats	93
Supraventricular arrhythmias	6
Sinus or junctional bradycardia	34
Second- or third-degree AV block	7

Ventricular fibrillation

Ventricular fibrillation is the rapid, totally incoordinate contraction of ventricular myocardial fibres. This is reflected in the ECG by irregular, chaotic electrical activity (Figure 11.1). Ventricular fibrillation causes circulatory arrest and unconsciousness develops within 10–20 s. Ventricular fibrillation is usually, but not always, initiated by an 'R on T' ventricular ectopic beat (Figure 11.2).

Ninety per cent of deaths caused by myocardial infarction are due to ventricular fibrillation. The incidence of fibrillation is highest in the first hour after the onset of chest pain and diminishes progressively thereafter. Forty per cent of deaths occur within the first hour. Thus many patients who are potentially treatable die before they can be admitted to hospital.

In those patients who reach hospital, however, ventricular fibrillation and other arrhythmias are sufficiently common to necessitate continuous ECG monitoring for 24–48 h in an area where facilities for resuscitation are immediately available, i.e. a coronary care unit.

Between 3 and 10% of patients with acute myocardial infarction develop ventricular fibrillation while in a coronary case unit. The main determinant of incidence of ventricular fibrillation in a coronary care unit is the delay before admission: the shorter the delay, the greater the incidence of ventricular fibrillation.

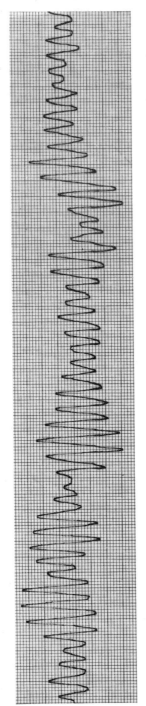

Figure 11.1 Ventricular fibrillation

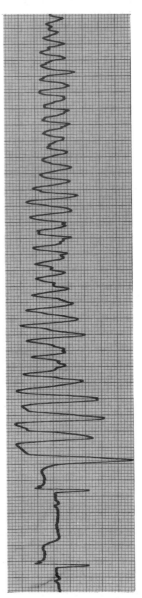

Figure 11.2. Ventricular ectopic beat initiating ventricular fibrillation

When ventricular fibrillation develops in a heart that was functioning satisfactorily during nomal rhythm it is termed 'primary' fibrillation, whereas if it occurs in the context of cardiac failure or cardiogenic shock, it is termed 'secondary'. Successful defibrillation is less likely in secondary ventricular fibrillation.

Ventricular fibrillation can occur without myocardial infarction in patients with severe coronary artery disease and may be the first clinical manifestation of the disease. Ventricular fibrillation can occur in other cardiac disorders but is discussed in this chapter because primary ventricular fibrillation due to myocardial infarction is a major cause of death in the Western world.

Rarely ventricular fibrillation is a brief event, spontaneously reverting to normal rhythm. Otherwise, without prompt treatment, irreversible cerebral and myocardial damage will quickly develop.

Treatment

Occasionally a praecordial blow is effective. Usually defibrillation is necessary (see Chapter 14). On a coronary care unit a defibrillator should be immediately available so that little or no time need be spent on cardiopulmonary resuscitation.

Successful defibrillation can be achieved with a 200 J DC shock in 90% of cases. If unsuccessful, a second shock at the same energy level may be effective. The energy of a further shock should be increased to 300 or 400 J. The treatment of resistant ventricular fibrillation is discussed in Chapter 14.

Once normal rhythm is restored, a lignocaine (or second-line drug if lignocaine has been found to be ineffective) infusion is given to prevent further ventricular fibrillation though it has to be said there is little evidence to show that lignocaine or other anti-arrhythmic drugs are effective in this situation.

Ventricular flutter

Ventricular flutter is a very fast ventricular rhythm in which there are rapid, continuous changes in waveform, distinction beween QRS complexes and T waves being impossible (Figure 11.3). For practical purposes, it is the same as ventricular fibrillation.

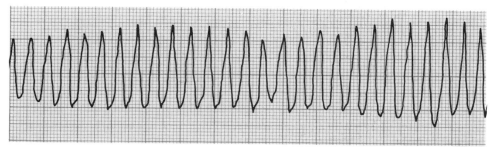

Figure 11.3 Ventricular flutter

Prevention of ventricular fibrillation

Conventional teaching used to be that ventricular fibrillation and tachycardia are heralded by ventricular ectopic beats which are frequent, multifocal, 'R on T', or are repetitive – 'the 'warning arrhythmias' (Figures 11.4–11.7). It was common practice to suppress these ectopic beats with anti-arrhythmic agents, usually lignocaine, in the hope that ventricular fibrillation will be prevented.

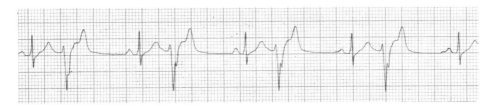

Figure 11.4 Frequent unifocal ventricular ectopic beats

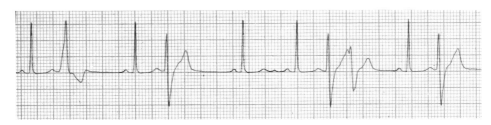

Figure 11.5 Frequent multifocal ventricular ectopic beats. The first ectopic beat arises from a different focus from that of subsequent ectopic beats. There is a couplet of ectopic beats after the fourth sinus beat

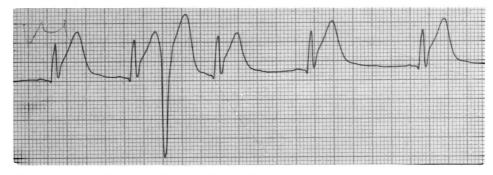

Figure 11.6 Interpolated 'R on T' ventricular ectopic beat

However, analysis of continuous ECG recordings has demonstrated that ventricular ectopic beats occur in virtually all cases of acute infarction and that warning arrhythmias are as common in patients who do not develop ventricular fibrillation as in those who do. Furthermore, there is evidence to show that ventricular fibrillation

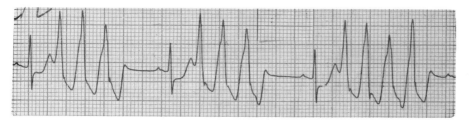

Figure 11.7 Salvoes of ventricular ectopic beats, initiated by 'R on T' ectopics

may not be preceded by warning arrhythmias and that when these do occur, staff in even the best coronary care units often fail to detect them.

Several studies have shown that there is an increased incidence of ventricular fibrillation if hypokalaemia is present but there is no evidence to indicate that a low serum potassum concentration is the direct cause of the arrhythmia.

It is disappointing that, in spite of 20 years of development in coronary care, there is no clear approach to the prevention of ventricular fibrillation. Until the situation is clarified by further studies one of two policies can be adopted:

1. *Prophylaxis for all patients with acute infarction* – This approach has been quite widely advocated on the grounds that since 'warning arrhythmias' do not in fact warn, lignocaine should be given to all patients with definite or suspected acute infarction. However, a consistently therapeutic plasma level of the drug is required. To achieve this, quite complex regimens of administration are necessary which may be impracticable for many busy coronary care units. Furthermore, with the high dosages of lignocaine that are required, side-effects due to lignocaine toxicity are frequent. Recently, it has been suggested that high doses of lignocaine may reduce the incidence of ventricular fibrillation only at the expense of a higher incidence of asystole. Reports vary as to whether lignocaine does actually reduce the incidence of ventricular fibrillation. With the possible exception of intravenous beta-blocking drugs, there are no reports of other drugs being of prophylactic value.

2. *No prophylaxis* – Since only a minority of patients develop ventricular fibrillation, some (including the author) advocate no prophylaxis provided trained staff are immediately available to defibrillate if ventricular fibrillation does occur. However, there are two reservations about this approach. First, occasionally it is not possible to resuscitate a patient with primary ventricular fibrillation. Secondly, though it is widely believed that the prognosis following correction of primary ventricular fibrillation is normal, there are a few reports suggesting that it may in fact be impaired.

Ventricular tachycardia

Ventricular tachycardia may be self-terminating (Figure 11.7) or sustained (Figure 11.8). Ventricular tachycardia may be initiated by either 'R on T' or late ventricular ectopic beats (Figure 11.9).

Sometimes ventricular tachycardia will result in shock or circulatory arrest. On the other hand, ventricular tachycardia may cause few or no syptoms. In myocardial

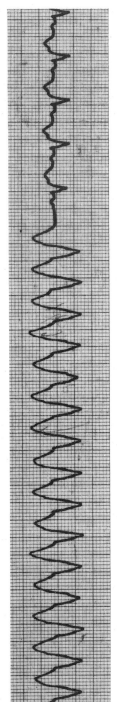

Figure 11.8 Ventricular tachycardia, terminated by mexiletine

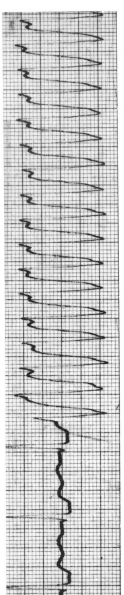

Figure 11.9 Ventricular tachycardia initiated by 'R on T' ectopic beat

infarction a regular tachycardia with broad ventricular complexes is usually ventricular in origin, even in the absence of haemodynamic deterioration (see Chapter 8).

Treatment

If cardiac arrest or shock occurs, immediate synchronized DC countershock is indicated. Otherwise intravenous lignocaine should be given. If lignocaine fails, second-line drugs include mexiletine, disopyramide, flecainide and amiodarone (see Chapter 12). Overdrive ventricular pacing should be considered in recurrent ventricular tachycardia or when a pacing wire is already in place for the treatment of a conduction disorder.

Long-term significance of ventricular arrhythmias

Early arrhythmias

Ventricular tachycardia and fibrillation that occur within the first 24 hours of myocardial infarction are unlikely to recur after that period. Furthermore, according to most studies, they are not related to the amount of myocardial damage sustained. Thus anti-arrhythmic therapy after discharge from the coronary care unit is not indicated and the arrhythmias are not of long-term prognostic significance.

Late arrhythmias

In contrast to early arrhythmias, ventricular tachycardia or fibrillation occurring more than 24–48 hours after infarction is likely to recur days, weeks or even months later. Long-term anti-arrhythmic therapy should be prescribed.

The more extensive the myocardial damage the worse the prognosis. Late ventricular arrhythmias are related to the size of the infarct. However, ventricular arrhythmias are also an independent predictor of prognosis, i.e. a patient with both extensive myocardial damage and late ventricular arrhythmias has a poorer prognosis than a patient with the same degree of myocardial damage but no arrhythmia (Table 11.2).

Table 11.2 Relation of ventricular tachycardia/fibrillation to infarct size and long-term treatment

	Related to infarct size	*Long-term treatment*
Early	Probably not	Not indicated
Late	Yes	Indicated

Though it clearly makes sense to prevent a recurrence of ventricular fibrillation or sustained ventricular tachycardia there is no evidence that suppression of ventricular ectopic beats or unsustained ventricular tachycardia improves prognosis.

Assessment of efficacy of long-term anti-arrhythmic therapy

Whatever treatment is chosen, it is important to ensure that it is effective in preventing a recurrence of the arrhythmia. It would seem logical to assume that the oral preparation of a drug which when given intravenously had restored normal rhythm would be effective in preventing a recurrence of arrhythmia. In practice, however, this is often not the case.

If the tachyarrhythmia or associated ventricular extrasystoles have been frequent then monitoring the electrocardiogram at the bedside or ambulatory electrocardiography are the best methods of assessing the efficacy of anti-arrhythmic therapy. In some cases where control has been difficult to achieve it may be necessary to accept a situation where ventricular extrasystoles and even short runs of ventricular tachycardia still occur – provided that the rate during tachycardia is significantly slower than before treatment.

If the arrhythmia has been an infrequent event then it is unlikely that ECG monitoring will reflect anti-arrhythmic control. Exercise ECG testing and electrophysiological testing (see Chapter 18) may be helpful.

Accelerated idioventricular rhythm

This is also referred to as idioventricular tachycardia or 'slow' ventricular tachycardia, is usually benign and treatment is not indicated (Figure 11.10). Rarely, acceleration of the rate can occur, necessitating treatment.

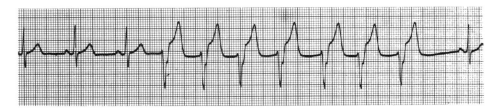

Figure 11.10 Accelerated idioventricular rhythm

Atrial ectopic beats

Occasional atrial ectopic beats can be ignored: however, frequent atrial ectopic beats often herald atrial fibrillation. It is best to digitalize the patient so that, should atrial fibrillation occur, the ventricular rate will be controlled.

Atrial fibrillation

In atrial fibrillation, the resultant rapid ventricular rate and reduction in cardiac output from loss of atrial systole can sometimes cause severe hypotension (see Figure 11.11). If shock occurs, immediate cardioversion may be necessary. Otherwise, the ventricular rate should be slowed by intravenous verapamil. If contraindicated, digoxin, a beta-blocker or amiodarone are alternatives. Spontaneous reversion to sinus rhythm is common.

Sustained atrial fibrillation is usually associated with extensive myocardial damage and/or older patients and hence a poor prognosis. Often there will be left ventricular

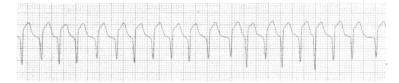

Figure 11.11 Atrial fibrillation with rapid ventricular rate in anterior infarction (lead V3)

failure in spite of control of the ventricular response to atrial fibrillation, necessitating diuretic therapy.

Paroxysmal supraventricular tachycardia

Paroxysmal (i.e. AV re-entrant) supraventricular tachycardia can only occur if there is an additional AV connection, either bypassing or within the AV node (see Chapter 6). Thus paroxysmal supraventricular tachycardia is unlikely to occur for the first time during acute myocardial infarction. When supraventricular tachycardia is diagnosed in a patient with acute infarction the correct diagnosis is usually atrial flutter, atrial fibrillation or even ventricular tachycardia.

Atrial flutter

The diagnostic features are discussed in Chapter 6. Usually 2:1 AV block occurs. Intravenous verapamil is useful, in that it will slow the ventricular rate and may occasionally effect a return to sinus rhythm. Low-energy DC countershock or rapid atrial pacing are often necessary for a prompt return to normal rhythm. Digoxin is best avoided because even large doses may not control the ventricular rate and will be a contra-indication to cardioversion.

Sinus and junctional bradycardias

Sinus and junctional bradycardias are common, particularly in inferior infarction (Figures 11.12 and 11.13). If uncomplicated, no treatment is required. Bradycardia may be beneficial in acute infarction, in that myocardial oxygen consumption is related to heart rate and a low oxygen consumption might limit infarct size.

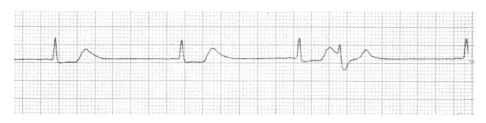

Figure 11.12 Sinus bradycardia. The fourth beat is an 'R on T' ventricular ectopic

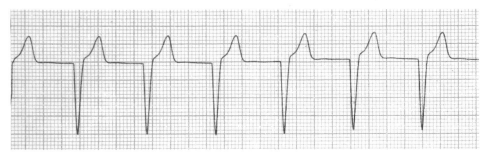

Figure 11.13 Junctional escape rhythm as a result of sinus bradycardia in anterior infarction (lead V4)

However, if bradycardia is associated with signs of low cardiac output such as hypotension (systolic blood pressure less than 90 mm Hg), mental confusion, oliguria, cold peripheries or ventricular arrhythmias, intravenous atropine (initially 0·3–0·6 mg) should be given. Temporary cardiac pacing is occasionally necessary and is preferable to frequent doses of atropine.

AV block

The management and prognosis of AV block in inferior and anterior infarction differ markedly.

Inferior infarction

In inferior infarction AV block is common and is often due to ischaemia of the AV node. Recovery of AV node function usually occurs within a few days although sometimes it takes up to 3 weeks. Permanent AV node damage is very rare. The prognosis for inferior infarction complicated by AV block is good.

First-degree and Mobitz type I second-degree (Wenkebach) AV block (Figures 11.14 and 11.5) require no treatment, although drugs that may worsen AV node function, e.g. digoxin and verapamil, should be avoided.

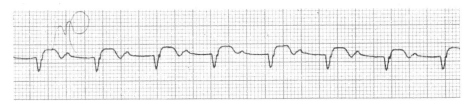

Figure 11.14 First-degree AV block (lead AVF)

If complete block develops (Figure 11.16), subsidiary pacemakers in the bundle of His control the ventricular rate. These pacemakers usually discharge at a fairly high rate. Thus asystole and symptoms resulting from a low ventricular rate are unusual.

However, sometimes the ventricular rate does fall very low (less than 40/min), when

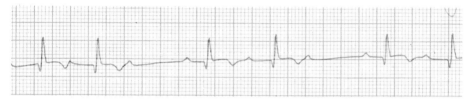

Figure 11.15 Wenkebach AV block in inferior infarction (lead AVF)

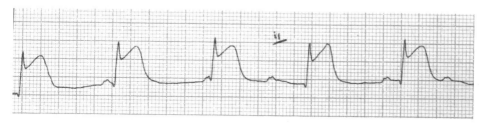

Figure 11.16 Inferior infarction complicated by complete AV block (lead II)

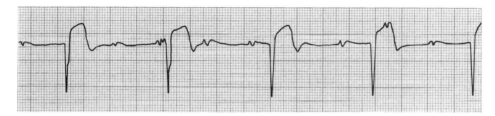

Figure 11.17 Complete heart block with ventricular rate of 38/min

Stokes–Adams attacks are likely to occur; or complications from a low ventricular rate such as heart failure, hypotension, mental confusion, oliguria and ventricular arrhythmias may result (Figure 11.17). In these circumstances temporary cardiac pacing is necessary. There is no place for steroids or catecholamines in an attempt to improve AV node function, although in the first 6 hours after infarction, atropine may be effective.

Sometimes AV block due to inferior infarction is a transient event and sometimes it can last for 2–3 weeks. AV block will almost always resolve within 3 weeks of infarction, and it is exceptional for long-term pacing to be necessary.

Anterior infarction

In anterior infarction it is the bundle branches rather than the AV node which are usually the site of ischaemic damage. AV block is more serious than in inferior infarction for two reasons. First, the subsidiary pacemakers which arise below the level of the block in the distal specialized conducting system tend to be slower and less reliable. Thus circulatory disturbances due to a low ventricular rate are common and ventricular standstill frequently occurs. Secondly, an extensive area of infarction is required to affect both bundle branches. Prognosis after myocardial infarction is related to the extent of infarction. Hence it is poor in patients with anterior infarction complicated by AV block.

Evidence of bilateral bundle branch damage (alternating right and left bundle branch block, or right bundle branch block with left anterior or posterior hemiblock) usually precedes the onset of second-degree (Mobitz type II) or complete AV block (Figures 11.18–11.21). The chance of bilateral bundle branch damage progressing to second-degree or complete heart block is approximately 30%. The first manifestation of these higher degrees of block may be ventricular standstill (Figure 11.22). For this reason a temporary transvenous pacemaker should be inserted when there is evidence of bilateral bundle branch damage even though the patient is in sinus rhythm.

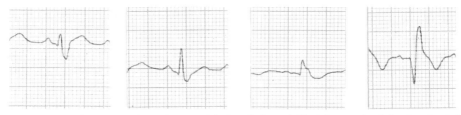

Figure 11.18 Left anterior fascicular and right bundle branch block in anterior infarction (leads I, II, III and V1)

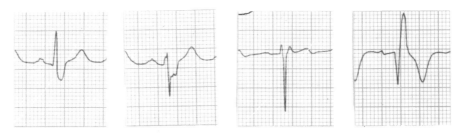

Figure 11.19 Left posterior fascicular and right bundle branch block in anterior infarction (leads I, II, III and V1)

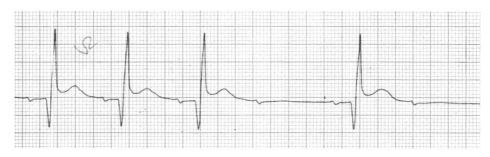

Figure 11.20 Intermittent Mobitz type II AV block in a patient with bifascicular block due to anterior infarction (lead V2)

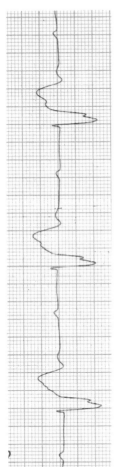

Figure 11.21 Complete AV block in a patient with anterior myocardial infarction. Because the atrial rate is twice the ventricular rate, at first glance in this short rhythm strip it appears that there is 2:1 AV block. However, measurement of the PR intervals indicates that they are not constant

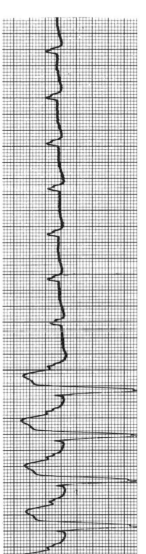

Figure 11.22 Sudden development of complete AV block in a patient with bifascicular block due to anterior infarction. Following four ventricular beats, there is asystole – only atrial activity is seen

Sometimes, bifascicular block has been present prior to acute infarction. In this situation the need for temporary pacing is less compelling.

Second- and third-degree AV block due to anterior infarction are always indications for temporary pacing. Sinus rhythm often returns after a few days but in some patients AV block will persist and may necessitate long-term pacing. Mortality is high in the first 3 weeks after anterior infarction complicated by AV block and long-term pacing should not be undertaken until the patient has survived this period.

If sinus rhythm does return, bifascicular block often persists. Complete AV block may recur in the weeks and months after acute infarction but there is no conclusive evidence to show that implantation of a pacemaker will improve prognosis. This is because the extensive myocardial damage associated with this situation will often lead to ventricular fibrillation or heart failure.

AV dissociation

In contrast to complete AV block, in AV dissociation the atrial rate is lower than the ventricular rate and no treatment is necessary.

Electrode placement for monitoring

Detection of atrial activity during an arrhythmia is often the key to the diagnosis. Chest electrodes for monitoring the ECG should be so placed that atrial activity can be clearly seen.

Lead V1 often shows atrial activity most clearly but is impracticable for continuous monitoring. A modified V1 lead can be achieved with three chest electrodes by placing the positive electrode over the fourth interspace at the right sternal edge, the negative electrode beneath the outer quarter of the left clavicle and the earth electrode beneath the outer quarter of the right clavicle. Not only will this lead system clearly show atrial activity, but it will allow distinction between beats having right and left bundle branch block appearance (Figure 11.23). In some patients, however, the lead system is not suitable because the ventricular complexes in lead V1 are of too small an amplitude.

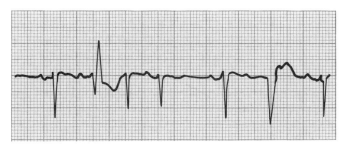

Figure 11.23 Modified V1 lead using three chest electrodes. Atrial ectopic beats conducted with right bundle branch block, normal intraventricular conduction and left bundle block can be seen

Main points

- Ventricular fibrillation occurs during the first hour of acute myocardial infarction in more than 30% of patients: the incidence falls progressively thereafter.

- Frequent, 'R on T' and other 'warning arrhythmias' are very common in acute infarction and are not predictive of ventricular fibrillation. Suppression by anti-arrhythmic drugs is not indicated.

- Immediate defibrillation should be carried out if ventricular fibrillation occurs.

- Ventricular fibrillation or other major ventricular arrhythmia during the first 24 hours of infarction is not an indication for long-term anti-arrhythmic therapy whereas therapy should be given if these arrhythmias occur after 24 hours.

- Atrial fibrillation, and ventricular arrhythmias arising 24 hours or more after acute infarction are usually associated with extensive myocardial damage and hence an impaired prognosis.

- Sinus and junctional bradycardia and complete AV block due to inferior infarction do not require treatment unless there are symptoms, marked hypotension, other signs of shock or ventricular arrhythmias.

- AV block due to acute inferior infarction may persist for up to 3 weeks and is very rarely an indication for permanent pacemaker implantation.

- In acute anterior infarction, a temporary pacemaker should be inserted if there is a second- or third-degree AV block or evidence of bilateral bundle branch damage. These conduction disturbances in the setting of anterior infarction imply extensive myocardial damage.

Chapter 12

Anti-arrhythmic drugs

Drugs are the mainstay of treatment for arrhythmias but their limitations should be appreciated.

Limitations of anti-arrhythmic drugs

- Limited efficacy
- Unwanted effects are common
- Difficulty in maintaining therapeutic drug levels
- Selection of an effective drug is often based on trial and error

First, anti-arrhythmic drugs are of limited effectiveness. In other words, a drug prescribed in the correct dose for an appropriate indication may fail to work.

Secondly, unwanted effects often occur. The most common are symptoms from the gastrointestinal and central nervous systems, hypotension, heart failure and impairment of the specialized cardiac conducting tissues. Occasionally, drugs may be 'pro-arrhythmic' in that they may worsen or cause arrhythmias.

Thirdly, with many drugs it may be difficult to maintain consistently therapeutic drug levels.

Fourthly, though considerable insight into the mode of action of anti-arrhythmic drugs has been gained, selection for an individual patient of a drug that is both effective and well tolerated is often a process of trial and error.

Drugs are only one form of treatment and in some situations other approaches such as vagal stimulation, cardioversion, artificial pacing, or surgery may be more appropriate. A number of factors may influence the choice of treatment: the type of arrhythmia, the urgency of the situation, the need for short- or long-term therapy, and the presence of impaired myocardial performance, sinus node dysfunction or abnormal AV conduction.

It is important to bear in mind why an anti-arrhythmic drug is being given. Sometimes, a drug is given to terminate an arrhythmia whereas at other times the purpose is prevention of its recurrence. Though it would seem reasonable to assume that the oral preparation of a drug that has terminated an arrhythmia when given intravenously would be successful in preventing its recurrence, this is often not the case in practice. Sometimes the aim of therapy is to slow the heart rate during the arrhythmia rather than to restore sinus rhythm. In some situations drugs are given to control symptoms whereas in others the purpose may be to prevent dangerous arrhythmias.

Modes of action

The modes of action of anti-arrhythmic drugs can be classified according to their effects in the intact heart (clinical classification) or according to their effects at cellular level as established by *in vitro* studies (action potential classification). The latter classification is widely referred to though it is of limited practical value.

Clinical classification

Drugs are divided into three groups according to their main site or sites of action in the intact heart:

Classification of anti-arrhythmic actions according to principal site(s) of action in intact heart

- AV node: Verapamil, diltiazem, digoxin, beta-blockers
- Ventricles: Lignocaine, mexiletine, tocainide, phenytoin
- Atria, ventricles and bundle of Kent: Quinidine, disopyramide, amiodarone, flecainide, procainamide, propafenone

The first group consists of drugs whose chief action is to slow conduction in the AV node. These drugs are therefore useful in the treatment of arrhythmias of supra-ventricular origin but are of little or no use in the treatment of ventricular arrhythmias.

   In the second group, there are drugs that work mainly in ventricular arrhythmias. The third group comprises drugs that act on the atria, ventricles and, in cases of Wolff–Parkinson–White syndrome, the bundle of Kent. Thus they may be useful in both supraventricular and ventricular arrhythmias.

Action potential classification

In this classification, drugs are divided into four main classes depending upon their electrophysiological effects at cellular level (Table 12.1).

Table 12.1 Examples of action potential classification

I		II	III	IV
A	Quinidine	Beta-blockers	Amiodarone	Verapamil
	Procainamide	Bretylium	Sotalol	Diltiazem
	Disopyramide		Bretylium	
	Pirmenol			
B	Lignocaine			
	Mexiletine			
	Tocainide			
	Phenytoin			
	Aprindine			
C	Flecainide			
	Encainide			
	Lorcainide			
	Propafenone			

   Class I drugs impede the transport of sodium across the cell membrane during the initiation of cellular activation and thereby reduce the rate of rise of the action potential (phase 0). Many drugs fall into this group. They have been subdivided into classes A, B and C according to their effect on the duration of the action potential (which is reflected in the surface electrocardiogram by the QT interval).

1A drugs increase the duration, 1B drugs shorten it and 1C drugs have little effect. The anti-arrhythmic action of 1B drugs is confined to the ventricles whereas 1A and 1C drugs affect both atria and ventricles. 1A and particularly 1C drugs slow intraventricular conduction.

Class II drugs interfere with the effects of the sympathetic nervous system on the heart. They do not affect the action potential of most myocardial cells but do reduce the slope of spontaneous depolarization (phase 4) of cells with pacemaker activity and thus the rate of pacemaker discharge.

Class III drugs prolong the duration of the action potential and hence the length of the refractory period, but do not slow phase 0.

Class IV drugs antagonize the transport of calcium across the cell membrane which follows the inward flux of sodium during cellular activation. Cells in the AV and sinus nodes are particularly susceptible. It should be noted that some calcium antagonists, e.g. nifedipine, do not have an anti-arrhythmic action.

Table 12.1 shows that the majority of drugs are in class I, some drugs have more than one class of action, and drugs within class I differ significantly in their clinical effects. Furthermore, some drugs, e.g. digoxin, cannot be classified.

Notes on individual drugs

Lignocaine

Lignocaine is the first-line drug for ventricular arrhythmias but is ineffective in arrhythmias of supraventricular origin. The drug is a vasoconstrictor and, unlike many drugs, rarely causes hypotension or heart failure.

A 100 mg bolus given intravenously over 2 min will usually be effective. If unsuccessful, a further bolus (50–75 mg) should be given after 5 min. There are several concentrations of lignocaine available, and disasters have occurred because the wrong concentration has been used. It should be remembered that 10 ml 1% lignocaine contains 100 mg.

Lignocaine is often used for short-term prophylaxis of ventricular arrhythmias. The therapeutic effect of lignocaine is closely related to plasma levels, which fall rapidly after a bolus injection. Thus it is necessary to give a continuous infusion immediately after the bolus. There is, however, no point in giving a continuous infusion if the bolus has failed to work or, since lignocaine cannot be administered by mouth, if long-term prophylaxis is required.

It can be difficult to maintain therapeutic levels of lignocaine. With sub-therapeutic levels, the patient is at risk from arrhythmias while toxic levels may cause symptoms related to the central nervous system, including light-headedness, confusion, twitching, paraesthesias and epileptic fits. With conventional infusion rates (1–4 mg/min) sub-therapeutic levels commonly occur in the first hour or two after the infusion is commenced. A number of fairly complex regimens have been developed to avoid this problem, though they may be too complex for routine use and do increase the risk of toxicity:

1. 75 mg i.v. bolus plus infusion at 10 mg/min for 20 min, reducing to 1·5 mg/min.
2. 25 mg/min up to total dose of 200–300 mg depending on body weight, followed by 2–3 mg/min.
3. Two 100 mg boluses separated by 10 min followed by infusion at 2–4 mg/min.

Lignocaine is metabolized by the liver, and where there is liver disease or where hepatic blood flow is reduced by heart failure or by shock, dosages should be halved to avoid toxicity. Hypokalaemia may impair lignocaine's efficacy.

Mexiletine

Mexiletine is similar to lignocaine in its therapeutic and haemodynamic actions but it can be given by mouth as well as parenterally. There is a narrow margin between therapeutic and toxic effects; and symptoms such as nausea, vomiting, confusion, tremor, ataxia, as well as bradycardia and hypotension, are not uncommon.

Intravenously, the drug is given in a dose of 100–250 mg over 5–10 min, followed by 250 mg over 1 h and a further 250 mg over 2 h. The infusion can then be continued at 0·5–1·0 mg/min or oral therapy started.

The oral dose is 200–300 mg 8-hourly. If the patient has not received a prior infusion, a loading dose of 400 mg can be given. Up to one-third of patients experience unwanted effects with long-term administration.

The drug is mainly metabolized by the liver and doses should be reduced if there is hepatic disease or heart failure. Approximately 10% is excreted unchanged in the urine. Renal excretion is inhibited by alkaline urine but this is not a problem in practice.

Though in the same anti-arrhythmic class as lignocaine, mexiletine may sometimes be effective when lignocaine has failed.

Tocainide

Tocainide is also similar to lignocaine. Like mexiletine it is effective both intravenously and by mouth. Its duration of action is somewhat longer than mexiletine, making twice daily oral administration possible. Forty per cent of the drug is excreted by the kidneys and dosage should be reduced if there is renal impairment.

The intravenous dosage is 750 mg over 15 min. The daily oral dosage is 1200 mg. Side-effects include tremor, light-headedness, confusion and convulsions.

Recently, there have been reports of tocainide causing agranulocytosis and thrombocytopenia. In the United Kingdom it is now recommended that the drug is only used for life-threatening ventricular arrhythmias where other drugs are ineffective or are contraindicated.

Quinidine

Quinidine can be effective in both supraventricular and ventricular arrhythmias. The drug is rarely used parenterally because severe hypotension may result. Orally, its use has been limited because of its reputation for causing dangerous rhythm disturbances, especially torsade de pointes tachycardia. However, slow-release preparations (e.g. Kinidin Durules) enable therapeutic levels to be maintained with much less risk of toxicity and have the advantage that twice-daily administration (0·5–0·75 g twice-daily) is sufficient.

Impaired sinus node and myocardial function are less likely to be worsened by quinidine than by disopyramide or beta-blockers. Because it has a mild anticholinergic action, AV node conduction may be enhanced with a resultant increase in ventricular rate during atrial flutter and fibrillation.

QT interval prolongation occurs with therapeutic doses, but lengthening of the

QRS complex by more than 25% indicates toxicity. The drug should not be given to patients whose QT interval is already prolonged. Gastrointestinal symptoms are not infrequent. Tinnitus, deafness, thrombocytopenia and hypotension occasionally occur. Quinidine therapy can elevate digoxin levels and precipitate toxicity. The drug is metabolized by the liver and doses should be reduced if there is hepatic disease.

Procainamide

Procainamide has similar anti-arrhythmic properties to quinidine. It is not widely used. It has a short half-life necessitating very frequent dosage when given by mouth. Even with a slow-release preparation, 8-hourly administration is necessary. Furthermore, unwanted effects such as systemic lupus syndrome, gastrointestinal symptoms, hypotension and agranulocytosis make it unsuitable for long-term use. Impaired renal function and a slow acetylator status both reduce procainamide requirements.

N-acetyl-procainamide, a metabolite of procainamide, has been shown to have a longer duration of action and not to cause systemic lupus.

Disopyramide

Disopyramide is widely used for both supraventricular and ventricular arrhythmias. However, it is only moderately effective and does have significant unwanted effects.

The intravenous dose is 1·5–2·0 mg/kg up to a maximum of 150 mh, given over no less than 5 min. The injection should be stopped if the arrhythmia is terminated. Therapy can be continued by intravenous infusion at 20–30 mg/h up to a maximum of 800 mg daily or the patient can be transferred to oral therapy. The oral dose is 300–800 mg daily in three or four divided doses. If necessary a loading dose of 300 mg can be given.

Given intravenously, the drug is more likely to cause hypotension and heart failure than lignocaine and related drugs and its use can be disastrous if the recommended minimum period of administration is ignored.

Orally, the drug's side-effects are mainly related to its anticholinergic (atropine-like) action which often causes a dry mouth, blurred vision, urinary hesitancy or retention and, by enhancing AV nodal conduction, an increase in the ventricular response to atrial flutter and fibrillation. The drug may precipitate heart failure in patients with impaired myocardial function. It may occasionally induce torsade de pointes tachycardia and should not be given to patients with QT interval prolongation. Disopyramide may worsen impaired sinus node function and is contraindicated in the sick sinus syndrome. The drug is partially excreted by the kidneys and dosage should be reduced in renal disease.

Flecainide

Flecainide is a potent drug which can be given both orally and parenterally. Its indications include ventricular arrhythmias and pre-excitation syndromes. It is very effective at suppressing ventricular ectopic beats but somewhat less so in the treatment of ventricular tachycardia.

It has a long half-life of approximately 16 hours which facilitates twice daily oral administration. The dosage is 100–200 mg twice daily. After a few days it may be possible to reduce the dosage. The intravenous dose is 2 mg/kg body weight over not less than 10 minutes, and because the drug has a significant negative inotropic effect, it should be given more slowly in patients with poor ventricular function. Flecainide is both metabolized by the liver and excreted by the kidney.

The drug has a narrow therapeutic range, i.e. it can be difficult to achieve a therapeutic action without unwanted effects. The most common side-effect is visual disturbance, particularly on rotating the head. Light-headedness and nausea can also occur. The drug has been shown to increase the endocardial pacing threshold.

The drug does have an important negative inotropic action and should be avoided in patients in heart failure or with extensive myocardial damage. It can be pro-arrhythmic, particularly in patients with a history of sustained ventricular tachycardia and/or poor ventricular function. In a recent study of patients with ventricular extrasystoles following myocardial infarction, flecainide was found to increase mortality.

Flecainide causes slight prolongation of the QRS complex and hence the QT interval: it does not prolong the JT component of the QT interval as does quinidine and disopyramide.

Amiodarone

This drug has several advantages over other drugs. It is highly effective in both supraventricular and ventricular rhythm disorders: even in arrhythmias refractory to other drugs there is a 70% success rate. It has a remarkably long half-life (20–100 days), so that the drug need only be given once daily or even less frequently. It does not significantly impair ventricular performance and can be given to patients in heart failure.

However, it has important unwanted effects which point to the long-term use of amiodarone being confined to patients with arrhythmias that are dangerous or resistant to other drugs, or where the risk of side-effects is not a major consideration because the patient's prognosis is poor, e.g. the elderly and those with severe myocardial damage.

The drug has a delayed onset of action. When given by mouth, it usually takes 3–7 days before it takes effect and it may take 50 days to achieve its maximal action. If necessary, delay can be minimized by giving large doses, e.g. 1200 mg daily for 1 or 2 weeks. The dose can then be reduced to 400–600 mg daily. Once the arrhythmia is controlled, it is recommended that the dose be progressively reduced until the lowest effective dose is found. The usual maintenance dose is 200–400 mg daily. In a few patients, a dose as small as 200 mg on alternate days will suffice. With dangerous arrhythmias where a recurrence cannot be risked, it is best not to reduce the dose below 400 mg daily.

The drug is thought to be metabolized by the liver. It is not excreted by the kidneys. The main metabolite is desethylamiodarone which may itself have an anti-arrhythmic action. Very high concentrations of amiodarone and its metabolite are achieved in the lungs, heart, liver and adipose tissue.

Intravenous administration will lead to an earlier effect than oral therapy but unlike most drugs, an immediate anti-arrhythmic effect rarely occurs: an effect is usually seen within 1–24 hours. When an arrhythmia has been difficult to control, it is often worth resorting to intraveous amiodarone in spite of possible delay in action rather than try further drugs which are less potent and which often cause unwanted effects.

The recommended intravenous dosage is 5 mg/kg body weight over 30 minutes to 1 hour followed by 15 mg/kg over 24 hours. In an emergency, the initial infusion can be given more rapidly but its vasodilator action may cause marked hypotension. It is important to give the drug via a central venous line to avoid phlebitis. If this is not possible, frequent changes of peripheral infusion site will often be sufficient.

Short-term treatment with intravenous amiodarone is unlikely to cause side-effects although recently two cases of hepatitis associated with the drug have been described.

Longer term oral therapy is associated with a high incidence of side-effects. The most common are corneal microdeposits and skin photosensitivity. Corneal micro-deposits occur in virtually all patients but ocular damage does not occur. The microdeposits disappear if the drug is stopped and are a useful sign of compliance. Skin photosensitivity to UV-A radiation affects over one third of patients and is the commonest reason for stopping the drug. It may persist for over a year afterwards. Though only a minority experience severe photosensitivity, all patients should be warned about the possibility. If necessary, protective clothing, avoidance of prolonged sunlight and barrier creams containing zinc oxide may be recommended.

Amiodarone contains iodine and causes elevation of both serum thyroxine and reversed tri-iodothyronine and depression of serum tri-iodothyronine. These changes are compatible with the euthyroid state. However, amiodarone can cause both hypothyroidism and hyperthyroidism. If the former occurs, serum thyroxine will be low and TSH will be elevated. Sometimes there will be no clinical signs of hypothyroidism. Thyroid hormone replacement is indicated. It is not essential to stop amiodarone. If hyperthyroidism occurs, the patient will often become unwell with weight loss and other signs of thyroid overactivity. Both serum thyroxine and tri-iodothyronine will be high. Amiodarone must be stopped and in severe cases short-term steroid therapy should be given.

Other serious side-effects include pulmonary alveolitis, hepatitis, neuropathy and myopathy. Pulmonary alveolitis is the most common of these problems. It usually presents with dyspnoea, which may be severe, and widespread shadowing in the lung fields which can be mistaken for pulmonary oedema. Amiodarone should be stopped and short-term therapy with steroids given. Sometimes several major unwanted effects occur together.

Patients receiving long-term amiodarone should have thyroid and liver function tests and chest X-rays at annual intervals. Usually but not invariably, serious side-effects are associated with higher dosages of amiodarone.

Other unwanted effects include nausea, rash, alopecia, tremor, insomnia and nightmares which can be very vivid. Long-term therapy may result in a characteristic blue–grey pigmentation of the skin. The drug's class III action results in QT prolongation, often with prominent U waves. There are a few reports of the drug causing torsade de pointes tachycardia.

It is important to note that the drug potentiates oral anticoagulants: usually halving the required dosage. Amiodarone increases blood levels of digoxin, quinidine and flecainide.

With many arrhythmias, the major advantages of amiodarone, its efficacy, absence of important negative inotropic action and long duration of action, are outweighed by the formidable list of side-effects. However, most of the side-effects are reversible and the risk of them should not be a contraindication in patients with life-threatening arrhythmias, a short life expectancy or in whom other anti-arrhythmic measures have failed.

Verapamil

Intravenous verapamil (5–10 mg over 30–60 s) quickly and effectively slows AV nodal conduction. It is the drug of choice for the termination of paroxysmal (AV re-entrant) supraventricular tachycardia. It will promptly slow the ventricular response to atrial fibrillation and flutter and in a minority of cases, in addition to its action on the AV node, may actually restore sinus rhythm.

Orally, verapamil is less effective and because much of each dose is metabolized by the liver, large doses (40 120 mg t.d.s.) are required. Verapamil by mouth is rarely useful alone but is very useful in combination with digoxin in controlling the ventricular response to atrial fibrillation if this cannot be achieved by apparently adequate doses of digoxin alone. Serum digoxin levels are in fact elevated by moderately large doses of verapamil.

Intravenous verapamil is contraindicated if the patient has received an intravenous or oral beta-blocker. Profound bradycardia or hypotension can result and may be fatal. Sometimes, the combination of oral verapamil and a beta-blocker will cause profound sinus or junctional bradycardia. Verapamil is contraindicated in patients with impaired sinus or atrioventricular node function or digoxin toxicity unless a ventricular pacing wire is *in situ* because of its depressant effects on the sinus and AV nodes.

Verapamil does have a significant negative inotropic effect and may cause hypotension in patients with very poor myocardial function. Two studies report that administration of intravenous calcium chloride immediately prior to parenteral verapamil prevents hypotension.

Beta-adrenoceptor antagonists

These drugs have anti-arrhythmic properties by virtue of their principal action – antagonizing the effects of catecholamines on the heart. They are most effective in arrhythmias caused by increased sympathetic nervous system activity, e.g. those caused by exertion, emotion, thyrotoxicosis, acute myocardial infarction and the hereditary QT prolongation syndromes.

Beta-blocking drugs slow AV nodal conduction and thus, like verapamil, are useful in arrhythmias of supraventricular origin. However, they are less often successful than verapamil, and, since the latter drug cannot be safely administered once beta-blockers have been given, verapamil is the treatment of choice. Unwanted bradycardia caused by beta-blockade can usually quickly be reversed by atropine.

Recently, a beta-blocker, esmolol, with an extremely short half-life of only two minutes has been introduced. Its beta-adrenoceptor antagonist action and any associated unwanted effects will therefore be brief.

Sotalol
Sotalol, in addition to its beta-blocking property, prolongs the duration of the action potential and hence QT interval: it has a significant class III, or amiodarone-like action. Unlike other beta-blockers, sotalol has a marked effect upon the recovery periods of atrial and ventricular myocardium and accessory AV pathways. Sotalol is more effective than other beta-blockers for prevention of supraventricular arrhythmias and may possibly be of value for ventricular arrhythmias. There are few reports of high doses of the drug   usually in association with other drugs or hypokalaemia   of causing torsade de pointes tachycardia. The oral dosage is 160–320 mg daily.

Digoxin

The main use of digoxin is as an AV nodal blocking drug in the control of the ventricular rate during atrial fibrillation. The usual dose is 0·25–0·375 mg daily. A number of factors – e.g. hypokalaemia, renal impairment, dehydration (often caused by diuretics) and therapy with quinidine, verapamil or amiodarone – predispose to digoxin toxicity and are an indication for dosage reduction.

Digoxin toxicity

Digoxin toxicity is a common problem. Over 10% of patients receiving the drug who are admitted to hospital have been found to have evidence of digoxin toxicity.

Several factors predispose to digoxin toxicity. These include impaired renal function, hypokalaemia, dehydration (often due to diuretics), age (the elderly are more susceptible to toxicity) and hypothyroidism. Quinidine, amiodarone and verapamil all increase digoxin levels.

A number of symptoms suggest digoxin toxicity. These include anorexia, nausea, vomiting, diarrhoea, mental confusion, xanthopsia and visual blurring. However, none of these symptoms is specific to digoxin toxicity; in patients with severe congestive heart failure in particular, gastrointestinal symptoms are often caused by heart failure rather than digoxin.

Digoxin toxicity can cause a number of disorders of cardiac rhythm. These include atrial tachycardia with AV block (Figure 12.1), junctional tachycardia (Figure 12.2), ventricular ectopic beats (often bigeminy) (Figure 12.3), ventricular tachycardia, first-, second- and third-degree AV block, a slow ventricular response to atrial fibrillation (Figure 12.4) and sino-atrial block (Figure 12.5).

The main use of digoxin is to control the ventricular rate during atrial fibrillation. When a patent receiving digoxin for this purpose develops a regular pulse a number of possibilities should be considered. First, sinus rhythm may have returned. Secondly, an arrhythmia due to digoxin toxicity may have developed, e.g. atrial tachycardia with AV block, junctional tachycardia or atrial fibrillation with complete AV block.

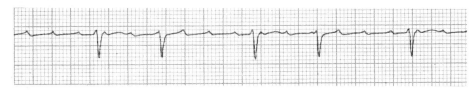

Figure 12.1 Atrial tachycardia with varying degrees of AV block

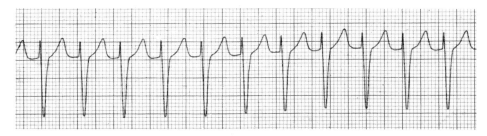

Figure 12.2 Junctional tachycardia

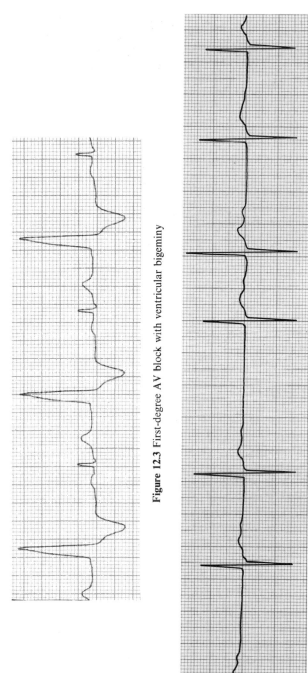

Figure 12.3 First-degree AV block with ventricular bigeminy

Figure 12.4 Slow ventricular response to atrial fibrillation

Figure 12.5 Junctional escape rhythm resulting from sinus arrest

Without an ECG it may be difficult to ascertain whether the regular rhythm is due to an arrhythmia or not.

Plasma digoxin levels can be measured but must be interpreted in conjunction with clinical features. Levels less than 1·5 ng/ml, in the absence of hypokalaemia, indicate that digoxin toxicity is unlikely. Levels in excess of 3·0 ng/ml indicate that toxicity is probable. With levels between 1·5 and 3·0 ng/ml digoxin toxicity should be considered a possibility, particularly if there are symptoms or arrhythmias attributable to digoxin toxicity or if there is renal impairment, or if the patient appears to be on an inappropriately large dose of digoxin. Blood for digoxin concentration estimation must be taken at least 6 hours after the last dose.

Usually temporary discontinuation of the drug and correction of hypokalaemia, if present, are all that is required. Serious ventricular arrhythmias should be treated with intravenous anti-arrhythmic drugs. Lignocaine is suitable, though animal studies suggest that Epanutin (phenytoin) may be preferable. It has also been suggested that beta-blockers are particularly effective; these, however, may worsen AV node function and increase the risk of AV block developing.

If high degrees of AV block occur, temporary cardiac pacing may be necessary. Cardioversion is dangerous in the presence of digoxin toxicity. If cardioversion is essential, low energy levels, e.g. 5–10 J, increasing gradually as necessary, should be used and lignocaine 75–100 mg should be given.

In cases of acute overdosage gastric lavage should be carried out. A temporary transvenous pacemaker should be inserted since there is a high likelihood of AV block developing. The heart rhythm should be monitored and arrhythmias treated accordingly.

Therapeutic range of plasma levels

The therapeutic range of plasma levels of the commonly used anti-arrhythmic drugs are given in Table 12.2. However, measurement of plasma levels is of limited use and is not often necessary in routine treatment.

If there is good evidence of a therapeutic effect with a standard dosage regimen and there are no unwanted effects, measurement of a drug's plasma level is of little importance. However, knowledge of a drug's level may be helpful with some clinical problems, e.g. when there is doubt as to whether a patient is taking his therapy or as to whether symptoms may be due to drug toxicity.

Table 12.2 Therapeutic range of plasma levels (μg/ml) for some anti-arrhythmic drugs

Amiodarone	1·0–2·5
Disopyramide	2·0–6·0
Flecainide	0·2–1·0
Lignocaine	1·4–6·0
Mexiletine	0·5–2·0
Procainamide	4·0–10·0
Quinidine	2·3–5·0
Tocainide	6·0–12·0
Verapamil	100–200

Main points

- Anti-arrhythmic drugs are of limited efficacy and often cause unwanted effects.

- Choice of anti-arrhythmic therapy should be tailored to the individual patient and depends on the arrhythmia, the degree of associated circulatory disturbance, the presence of impaired myocardial, sinus node or AV node function, need for short- or long-term treatment and concurrent adminis-tration of other drugs.

- Drugs are usually better at terminating arrhythmias than at preventing their recurrence.

- Intravenous verapamil should not be given to a patient who has received a beta-blocker.

- Disopyramide, flecainide and beta-blockers have a marked negative inotropic action and may precipitate heart failure in patients with extensive myocardial damage.

- Intravenous verapamil is the drug of choice for the acute control of arrhythmias of supraventricular origin.

- Lignocaine is the first-line drug for termination of ventricular tachycardia.

- Amiodarone is the most effective anti-arrhythmic agent currently available but its long-term use should be confined to the treatment of patients with arrhythmias that are dangerous or are refractory to other forms of treatment, or who have a poor prognosis.

Chapter 13

Cardioversion

Cardioversion is the use of an electric shock of high energy and brief duration to terminate a tachyarrhythmia. The shock, which is usually delivered by two electrodes placed on the chest wall, depolarizes the myocardium thus interrupting the tachycardia and allowing the sinus node to resume control of the heart rhythm.

Procedure

Facilities for monitoring the ECG and for cardiopulmonary resuscitation must be available. The rhythm should be checked immediately prior to cardioversion to ensure that spontaneous reversion has not occurred.

Anaesthesia

Cardioversion is painful, causing involuntary contractions of the chest wall and upper limb girdle muscles. A conscious patient should be given a short-acting anaesthetic, or at least an amnesic agent, e.g. intravenous midazolam or intravenous diazepam. The patient should fast for 6 h before elective cardioversion, though this will not be possible in an emergency.

Delivery of shock

The shock is delivered by means of two electrode paddles placed on the chest wall, positioned so that the heart lies between them. Usually one electrode is placed over the cardiac apex and the other to the right of the upper sternum. Alternatively, if a flat paddle is available this can be placed beneath the patient's back, behind the heart, and the second paddle positioned anteriorly over the praecordium.

To achieve good electrical contact and to avoid burning the skin, electrode jelly must be generously applied to the areas beneath the paddles. However, it is essential to avoid spreading jelly between the two paddles. Recently, pads impregnated with electrode gel have been introduced, with the advantage that they avoid the spreading of jelly over unwanted areas, including the operator!

The defibrillator is charged to the desired energy level (see below), which takes a few seconds. The charge is usually released by pressing the button(s) on the defibrillator paddle(s). Application of the paddles with firm pressure reduces the electrical resistance of the thorax. Before discharge it is essential to ensure that no one is in contact with the patient or the patient's bed.

If cardioversion is unsuccessful, depending on the circumstances, further shocks with higher energy levels may be tried. The heart rhythm should usually be monitored for a few hours after cardioversion.

Synchronization

Ventricular fibrillation may be induced if a shock coincides with the ventricular T wave. For this reason, most defibrillators have a synchronizing mechanism whereby discharge is triggered to occur at the time of the R or S wave. The synchronizing mechanism should be used during cardioversion for all arrhythmias with the exception of ventricular fibrillation. With ventricular fibrillation there will be no detectable R wave and thus, if the synchronizing mechanism is in operation, the defibrillator will not discharge. Before synchronized cardioversion, the operator should check that the synchronizing signal coincides with the onset of the QRS complex. Sometimes, the amplitude of the ECG has to be increased to enable synchronization.

Energy levels

In general, low energy levels are used initially. If unsuccessful, further shocks can be given at increased levels. The initial energy setting depends on clinical circumstances. For example, atrial flutter usually responds to low-energy shocks – 25 J would be an appropriate initial level. On the other hand, with ventricular fibrillation it is best to use a fairly high level – 200 J initially. When digoxin toxicity is suspected, very low levels should be used, starting at 5–10 J. For other arrhythmias it is usual to start at 50 s and increase by increments of 50–100 J. Levels of 400 J should not be exceeded.

In children lower energy levels should be used, starting at 5–10 J.

Complications

Complications are rare. Hypotension and heart failure are occasionally produced. Enzyme levels are elevated in some patients and may be due to either skeletal or cardiac muscle damage. Transient arrhythmias are sometimes induced by cardioversion but these are rarely a problem unless there is digoxin toxicity. In patients with the bradycardia–tachycardia syndrome a profound bradycardia may be caused by cardioversion. When this syndrome is suspected a temporary pacing wire should be inserted before cardioversion. Systemic embolism may occur when cardioversion is carried out for arrhythmias of supraventricular origin (see below).

Nitrate patches or paste should be removed from the chest to avoid the risk of explosion.

Digoxin toxicity

Cardioversion in the presence of digoxin toxicity can produce dangerous ventricular arrhythmias. For this reason cardioversion should be used as a last resort when there is digoxin toxicity and should be preceded by lignocaine 75–100 mg. Because of the dangers of digoxin toxicity, it has become common practice to discontinue digoxin for 24–48 h prior to cardioversion in all cases. However, cardioversion in the presence of therapeutic levels of digoxin is safe. Cardioversion need not be postponed if one can be quite certain that digoxin toxicity is not present, i.e. the dose of digoxin is not excessive, renal function and plasma electrolytes are normal and there are no symptoms or ECG findings suggestive of digoxin toxicity.

Anticoagulation

In patients with atrial fibrillation or flutter, thrombus may develop in the atria and be dislodged when sinus rhythm returns. For this reason anticoagulation should be given before elective cardioversion when the cause of the arrhythmia is associated with a significant risk of systemic embolism, i.e. mitral valve disease, bradycardia–tachycardia syndrome and acute thyrotoxicosis. Oral anticoagulants should preferably be started 3 weeks before cardioversion and should be continued for 3 weeks afterwards.

Implanted pacemaker

Cardioversion may cause pacemaker damage but this should be prevented if the paddles are at least 15 cm from the generator and preferably are positioned so they are at right angles to the pacing system. Pacemaker function should be checked after the procedure.

Indications

Ventricular fibrillation

Rarely, a praecordial blow will effect a return to sinus rhythm; otherwise, immediate cardioversion is indicated. The initial energy level should be 200 J. If unsuccessful, a further 200 J shock should be given. If restoration of normal rhythm has still not been achieved a 400 J shock should be delivered.

Ventricular tachycardia

Cardioversion should be carried out if the arrhythmia has caused shock or cardiac arrest, or if drug therapy has failed.

Atrial fibrillation

Cardioversion usually effects a return to sinus rhythm. The problem, however, is that atrial fibrillation returns in a high proportion of patients within a few months and often within hours of cardioversion. A long-term successful result is more likely when cardiomegaly, left atrial enlargement and a long history of the arrhythmia are absent. Treatment with quinidine, disopyramide or amiodarone has been shown to increase modestly the chances of sinus rhythm being maintained.

Atrial flutter

This arrhythmia, which is often difficult to treat with drugs, responds to low energy shocks. The initial setting should be 25 J.

Paroxysmal supraventricular tachycardia

Cardioversion is indicated on the occasions when other measures, such as vagal stimulation or intravenous verapamil, have failed.

Main points

- The usual positions for the defibrillator paddles are the cardiac apex and to the right of the upper sternum. Firm pressure should be applied to the paddles when the DC shock is delivered.

- With the exception of ventricular fibrillation, delivery of the shock should be synchronized to the R or S wave of the electrocardiogram.

- Initial energy levels depend on the clinical circumstances: 25 J for atrial flutter, 200 J for ventricular fibrillation, 50–100 J for most other arrhythmias.

- Digoxin toxicity is a contraindication to cardioversion. Temporary transvenous pacing should be used to cover cardioversion if the bradycardia–tachycardia syndrome is suspected.

- In patients with atrial fibrillation or flutter due to conditions associated with a significant risk from systemic embolism, oral anticoagulation for 3 weeks should precede cardioversion.

- Damage to an implanted pacemaker can be prevented if the paddles are placed at least 15 cm from the generator and preferably positioned so they are at right angles to the pacing system.

Chapter 14

Cardiac arrest

Cardiac arrest is the cessation of an effective cardiac output as the result of a sudden circulatory or respiratory catastrophe. Patients dying from terminal and irreversible diseases will not benefit from and should not undergo the indignity of cardiopulmonary resuscitation.

Common causes

1. Acute myocardial infarction.
2. Severe coronary artery disease.
3. Anoxia, e.g. due to drowning, smoke inhalation, airways obstruction, or respiratory depression.
4. Electrocution.
5. Iatrogenic, e.g. hypokalaemia, or overdose of opiate or catecholamine.
6. Anaphylactic response to a drug or other allergen.

Diagnosis

Diagnosis of cardiac arrest is based on only two signs:

1. Unconsciousness.
2. Absent carotid or femoral artery pulsation.

Time should not be wasted in eliciting other signs of cardiac arrest such as dilated pupils, apnoea, and absent heart sounds.

Cardiopulmonary resuscitation

Management of cardiac arrest can be divided into three stages:

1. Basic life support.
2. Restoration of spontaneous heart action.
3. After-care.

Speed and efficiency in both the diagnosis and management of cardiac arrest are essential. The shorter the delays in starting basic life support and in restoring normal heart action, the more likely is a successful outcome.

Basic life support

This term refers to the combination of external chest compression and expired air respiration. Equipment and drugs are not required.

External chest compression

The heel of one hand is placed over the sternum at the junction of its upper two-thirds and lower one-third and is covered by the other hand. Keeping the arms straight, and with the shoulders directly aligned above the hands, the sternum should be depressed 4–5 cm at a rate of 80 beats per minute. Each compression should be sustained so that the time spent in compression is equal to that of relaxation.

If there is only one rescuer, after each 15 compressions, there should be a pause to deliver two expired air inflations. If there are two rescuers, after each five compressions there should be a pause for one expired air inflation. It is not necessary to use all one's force in compression; a flail chest or visceral damage may result.

Chest compression was thought to work by squeezing the ventricles between the sternum and vertebrae thereby expelling blood into the arteries. Hence the older term 'cardiac massage'. However, it is now known that chest compression increases intrathoracic pressure and thereby propels blood into the systemic arteries. Regurgitation into the venous system is prevented by valves at the superior thoracic inlet and, between chest compressions, the aortic valve remains competent, thus preventing blood flowing back into the heart. One piece of evidence that supports the view that the heart is a passive conduit during chest compression may be of practical value: rapid, vigorous coughing at the onset of ventricular fibrillation may generate sufficient cardiac output to maintain consciousness.

Expired air respiration

With the palm of one hand the patient's head should be tilted backwards so that the neck is fully extended. With the fingers of the other hand the lower jaw should be lifted forward so that it protrudes beyond the upper teeth. Without these manoeuvres the tongue will obstruct the airway and artificial ventilation will be impossible.

Mouth-to-mouth respiration should then be given by taking a deep breath and, after pinching the patient's nose and sealing the lips around those of the patient, blowing forcefully into the patient's mouth. The patient's chest should be seen to rise, otherwise ventilation is inadequate. If chest expansion is not achieved, the pharynx should be examined to ensure that it is not obstructed by vomit or foreign material.

As stated above, with one operator two ventilations should be given after each 15 chest compressions. With two operators, each five compressions should be followed by one ventilation.

If first attempts at restoring normal heart action (see below) are unsuccessful, an endotracheal tube should be inserted.

Restoration of normal heart action

Treatment depends on the heart rhythm. The paddles of a modern defibrillator also function as electrodes, enabling the heart rhythm to be quickly ascertained.

The ECG may reveal ventricular fibrillation, ventricular tachycardia, asystole or, very rarely, sinus rhythm. The latter may occur as a result of electrochemical dissociation, massive pulmonary embolism or cardiac tamponade, e.g. due to a ruptured left ventricle.

Ventricular fibrillation

Occasionally, a single blow to the praecordium with the side of a clenched first will, if given shortly after the onset of ventricular fibrillation (or tachycardia), restore sinus rhythm.

Otherwise, the patient should be immediately defibrillated. Time should not be wasted with basic life support procedures if a defibrillator is to hand. To avoid one common cause of delay, it is important to ensure familiarity with the controls of the available defibrillator(s).

The defibrillator should be charged to 200 J. One paddle should be firmly applied to the right of the upper sternum and the other to the cardiac apex after having placed electrode jelly or pads impregnated with electrode gel beneath the paddles. Everyone should be instructed to avoid contact with the patient who is then defibrillated by depressing the button(s) on the defibrillator paddle(s). Trinitrin patches or paste should be removed before defibrillation to avoid any risk of explosion.

If an arterial pulse is not palpable within 3 s of defibrillation, 15 chest compressions should be administered and then the heart rhythm ascertained. If ventricular fibrillation persists, a further 200 J shock should be given.

The majority of episodes of ventricular fibrillation will be terminated by the first or second 200 J shock. If the second attempt at defibrillation is unsuccessful a shock of 300–400 J should be given after a further 15 chest compressions. When ventricular fibrillation persists, further action is detailed in the summary below.

Summary of sequence of actions whilst ventricular fibrillation persists

1. 200 J shock.
2. 200 J shock.
3. 400 J shock.
4. Lignocaine 100 mg.
5. 400 J shock.
6. Adrenaline 5–10 ml of 1:10 000.
7. 400 J shock.
8. Sodium bicarbonate 50 ml 8·4%.
9. 400 J shock.

The purpose of adrenaline is to increase peripheral resistance and thereby divert blood flow to the myocardium. Experiments in animals suggest that this facilitates defibrillation though recent observations in man suggest that adrenaline may possibly have a deleterious effect. Sodium bicarbonate used to be given in large doses at the start of cardiopulmonary resuscitation to reverse acidosis but it is now appreciated that this practice is not necessary and may be harmful. Hence, adrenaline and sodium bicarbonate should be reserved for resistant ventricular fibrillation.

Ventricular tachycardia

If there is ventricular tachycardia it is preferable to set the synchronizing mechanism so that the shock falls on the R wave rather than the T wave to avoid the risk of inducing ventricular fibrillation. If the synchronization button is depressed it will not be possible to deliver a shock during ventricular fibrillation since no R waves will be detected.

Asystole

Resuscitation from asystole is often successful when the cause is anoxia or disease confined to the specialized conducting tissues. In the former case ventilation may be all that is required. In the latter case the mechanical stimulation of repeated praecordial blows or cardiac massage may initiate ventricular activation and maintain a satisfactory cardiac output. On the other hand, when asystole is due to extensive myocardial damage the prognosis is poor.

When ventilation and mechanical stimulation are ineffective, atropine 1·0 mg is occasionally effective. Otherwise 5–10 ml 1:10 000 adrenaline should be given. Further doses of adrenaline may be necessary – the asystolic heart can tolerate large doses of catecholamines. Defibrillation is useless in asystole.

Occasionally ventricular standstill may occur during atrial fibrillation and be confused with fine ventricular fibrillation. Pacing is rarely effective unless asystole is due to disease of the specialized conducting tissues.

Sinus rhythm

If cardiac arrest is thought to be due to cardiac tamponade, immediate aspiration of the pericardium or thoracotomy is indicated. Where pulmonary embolism is suspected, 15 000 units heparin should be given intravenously. If facilities are to hand, emergency pulmonary embolectomy may be possible.

In patients with myocardial damage dissociation between electrical and mechanical activity can sometimes be reversed with intravenous calcium chloride and adrenaline.

Administration of drugs

Drugs given via a peripheral vein during cardiac arrest may not reach the heart. Instead, a line should be inserted into a central vein. The femoral vein is a good approach, since it is remote from the area of resuscitation. The external jugular vein is often distended during cardiac arrest, allowing easy cannulation. In some patients it may be necessary to cannulate the internal jugular or subclavian vein.

If a venous line cannot be established, adrenaline and lignocaine can be given via the intrapulmonary route. They should be diluted in 10 ml saline and be given through a fine catheter, introduced via the endotracheal tube, deep into the lungs. Doses should be double those used intravenously.

As a last resort intracardiac injection may be carried out. A long fine needle should be introduced either at the apex and advanced towards the right shoulder or through the fourth left intercoastal space, lateral to the sternum, until blood is aspirated.

After-care

The patient should be transferred to an intensive care unit. The heart rhythm should be monitored during transfer. If cardiac arrest was due to ventricular fibrillation or tachycardia, lignocaine or a second-line anti-arrhythmic agent should be given.

In patients who have been asystolic, unless there has been a readily reversible cause, e.g. anoxia, a temporary pacemaker should be inserted.

When there is impaired consciousness, intravenous dexamethasone (8 mg) and frusemide should be given to relieve cerebral oedema. Artificial ventilation may be necessary as may be inotropic drugs.

The blood acid–base state should be checked by analysis of arterial blood withdrawn from the femoral or radial artery. Severe acidosis should be reversed by giving 8·4% sodium bicarbonate using the formula: ml required = body weight (kg) × 0·2 × base deficit.

Out-of-hospital sudden cardiac death

Sudden death due to cardiac disease is common. The annual incidence in the United Kingdom has been estimated to be 50 000. The mechanism is usually ventricular tachycardia of fibrillation. Ventricular fibrillation often results from degeneration from ventricular tachycardia rather than being the primary arrhythmia.

Coronary heart disease is by far the most common cause. Though acute myocardial infarction commonly leads to ventricular fibrillation, it accounts for less than one-third of patients presenting with sudden death. The majority have been found to have extensive coronary disease and poor left ventricular but not acute infarction. Other causes include dilated and hypertrophic cardiomyopathies, myocarditis, Wolff–Parkinson–White syndrome and hereditary prolongation of the QT interval.

Several centres, mainly in North America, have shown that facilities for out-of-hospital cardiopulmonary resuscitation do save lives. As a result, information on the syndrome of 'aborted sudden cardiac death' is increasing. It is now clear that patients who are resuscitated and who have not sustained acute infarction remain at risk. There is a recurrence rate of up to 60% within 2 years.

Patients resuscitated from cardiac arrest not caused by acute infarction must be investigated to assess the need for myocardial revascularization, anti-arrhythmic drug therapy or implantation of an automatic defibrillator before discharge from hospital.

The role of drugs is usually assessed by electrophysiological testing. It is usually possible to induce ventricular tachycardia in patients with 'aborted sudden cardiac death' by stimulating the heart with precisely timed premature ventricular stimuli. Drug therapy which then prevents re-induction of the arrhythmia or at least increases the cycle length during tachycardia by over 100 ms has been shown to have a very favourable effect on prognosis. Serial testing may be required to identify an effective drug. Sometimes all anti-arrhythmic drugs will be found to be ineffective. The implantable defibrillator has the advantage of being very effective in limiting mortality but currently available devices have disadvantages as outlined in Chapter 5.

Main points

- Loss of consciousness plus absence of carotid or femoral artery pulsation are the only signs required for the diagnosis of cardiac arrest.

- Chest compression is often poorly performed. Precise positioning of the hands, at the junction of the upper two-thirds and lower-third of the sternum, is essential. The operator's arms should be kept straight by 'locking the elbows', with the shoulder positioned directly above the hands. The chest should be compressed at a rate of 80 beats per minute, the duration of each compression should be sustained and equal to the relaxation phase.

- Maintenance of a clear airway by full extension of the neck is essential for effective mouth-to-mouth resuscitation.

- If there is ventricular fibrillation, the sooner defibrillation is carried out the more likely a successful outcome. Initially, 200 J should be delivered, the two paddles being positioned at the cardiac apex and to the right of the upper sternum. To avoid one common cause of delay, there should be familarity with the controls of the defibrillator(s) that one is likely to use.

- Out of hospital sudden cardiac death is usually due to ventricular tachycardia or fibrillation resulting from coronary heart disease. Frequently, there will be no evidence of acute myocardial infarction: without treatment recurrence is likely.

Chapter 15

Temporary cardiac pacing

Indications

The most common indications for temporary cardiac pacing are as follows.

Stokes–Adams attacks

As a first-aid measure in patients who present with syncope or near-syncope due to chronic disease of the sinus node or AV junction who require long-term pacing.

Acute myocardial infarction (see Chapter 11)

Bifascicular, second- and third-degree AV block due to acute anterior myocardial infarction.

Second- or third-degree AV block caused by acute inferior infarction which is complicated by hypotension, heart failure, ventricular tachyarrhythmia or ventricular rate less than 40 beats per minute.

Symptomatic sinus arrest or junctional bradycardia due to acute myocardial infarction.

General anaesthesia

Patients with second- or third-degree AV block should have a pacemaker to cover the operative period. They may subsequently require long-term pacing.

In the absence of a history of syncope or near-syncope, the risk of AV block developing during anaesthesia in a patient with bifascicular block is very low and pacing is not essential.

Tachycardias

Pacing is useful in terminating paroxysmal supraventricular tachycardia, atrial flutter and ventricular tachycardia. In the bradycardia–tachycardia syndrome temporary pacing should be used to cover cardioversion if required for the termination of supraventricular arrhythmias.

Methods

The transvenous route is usually used for temporary pacing but, in emergencies, transcutaneous and oesophageal approaches are possible short-term alternatives.

Temporary transvenous pacing

Temporary ventricular pacing is usually carried out by introducing a transvenous pacing electrode under local anaesthesia into a systemic vein and advancing it, with the aid of X-ray screening, to the right ventricle. The electrode is connected to an external battery-powered pulse generator. During insertion the heart rhythm must be monitored and equipment for resuscitation should be available. A recent survey has demonstrated that this essentially simple procedure frequently leads to complications when carried out by inexperienced, unsupervised operators.

Subclavian vein puncture

The subclavian vein is the most suitable route of access to the venous system. The vein runs behind the medial third of the clavicle and can be punctured using either supraventricular or infraclavicular approaches. Only the latter will be described.

The patient should be laid flat or, if possible, in a slight head-down position. A needle is introduced, through a $\frac{1}{2}$-cm skin incision, just below the inferior border of the clavicle, slightly medial to the mid-clavicular point, and is directed towards the sternoclavicular joint so that it passes immediately behind the posterior surface to the clavicle. When first advancing the needle it is advisable to locate the clavicle with the needle to avoid going in too deeply, with consequent risk of pneumothorax or subclavian artery puncture.

As the needle punctures the vein, venous blood will be easily aspirated. If there is only a trickle of blood the needle tip is unlikely to be in the subclavian vein.

Cannulation of the vein is best achieved by introducing a guide wire through the needle into the vein. A guide wire with a flexible J-shaped tip is much easier to advance around the junction between the subclavian vein and superior vena cava, which can often be quite an acute bend. The needle is then withdrawn and a sheath within which there is a vessel dilator is passed over the wire into the vein. The guide wire and dilator are then removed, and the pacing lead is passed through the sheath. It is important to ensure before vein puncture that the lead will easily pass through the sheath.

The main advantages of subclavian vein puncture are that it is quick and infection and electrode displacement are unusual. Possible complications, which are rare in experienced hands, are pneumothorax, haemothorax, subclavian artery puncture and air embolism.

Antecubital vein cut-down

It is important to select a medially situated vein. It is unusual to be able to negotiate an electrode into the superior vena cava from a lateral vein.

The disadvantages of this method are that electrode stability is poor, even when the patient's arm is strapped to his side, and infection and phlebitis are not uncommon.

Femoral vein puncture

This method is very easy and quick, provided that pulsation of the laterally adjacent femoral artery is easily palpable. However, it should be reserved for short-term emergency purposes because electrode stability is poor and there is a risk of venous thrombosis. Pressure on the abdomen causes distension of the femoral vein and makes venepuncture easier.

Positioning of the electrode

If there is resistance to the introduction of the electrode into the vein, the lumen has probably not been entered. Once in the venous system, it should be possible to advance the electrode without any resistance. If an obstruction is encountered, the electrode should be withdrawn slightly, rotated and then advanced again. Nothing will be achieved by forcing the electrode.

Once the electrode has reached the right atrium, a loop should be formed by impinging the electrode tip on the atrial wall (Figure 15.1A) and then advancing the electrode a little further (Figure 15.1B). By twisting the electrode, the loop is then rotated so that the electrode tip lies near the tricuspid valve (Figure 15.1C). Slight withdrawal of the electrode will allow the tip to 'flick' through the valve into the right ventricle.

Ventricular ectopic beats are usually provoked as the valve is crossed. If these do not occur the coronary sinus rather than the right ventricle may have been entered. An electrode lying in the coronary sinus assumes a characteristic shape (Figure 15.1F). (A lateral view will show that the electrode is pointing posteriorly whereas an electrode in the right ventricular apex points anteriorly.) It can be confirmed that the right ventricle has been entered by advancing the electrode into the pulmonary artery (Figure 15.1D).

Once in the right ventricle, the electrode tip is positioned in or near the apex of the ventricle by a process of advancement, withdrawal and rotation (Figure 15.1E).

Difficulty with electrode manipulation can be due to poor technique. Another cause is that reusable pacing electrodes lose their stiffness after repeated use and should not be employed more than six times. If positioning proves difficult, it is well worth trying a new electrode.

Pacing

When a stable electrode position in or near the right ventricular apex has been achieved, the distal and proximal poles of the electrode should be connected to the pacemaker cathode ($-$) and anode ($+$), respectively. If the poles are connected the other way round, the stimulation threshold will be substantially higher. The pacing threshold, which is the minimum voltage necessary for pacing stimuli to capture the ventricles consistently, should then be measured (Figure 15.2). It should be less than 1·0 V (assuming that the temporary pacemaker delivers impulses whose duration is 2 ms. Some temporary pacemakers allow the pulse width to be adjustable: shorter pulse widths will lead to a higher threshold and are virtually never indicated for temporary pacing.) If not, the electrode should, if possible, be repositioned.

Sometimes, particularly in an emergency, a pacing threshold or electrode position which is less than optimal has to be accepted. Occasionally a patient may become dependent on the pacemaker, making adjustment of the electrode position hazardous.

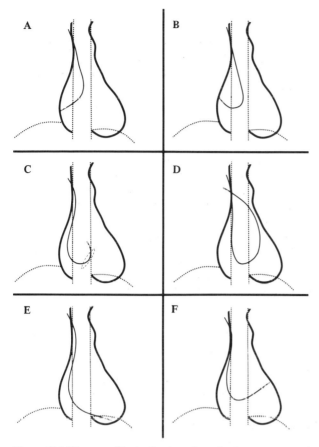

Figure 15.1 Diagrams illustrating insertion of a transvenous pacing lead. A loop is formed in the right atrium (A and B). The loop is positioned near the tricuspid valve, indicated by the oval of dashes (C). Entry into the right ventricle can be confirmed by passing the wire into the pulmonary artery (D). The pacing lead is then positioned in the apex of the right ventricle (E). (F) The characteristic appearance of a pacing lead in the coronary sinus

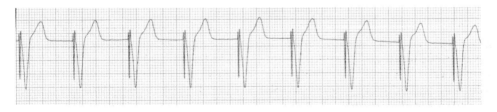

Figure 15.2 Ventricular pacing (lead II). Each pacing stimulus is followed by a ventricular complex. An electrode positioned in the apex of the right ventricle will produce left axis deviation of the paced beats

In these circumstances it may be necessary to insert a second pacing electrode (e.g. via the femoral vein) to cover the period of repositioning.

The stability of the pacing lead should be tested by ensuring that there is consistent pacing during coughing and deep inspiration. During the latter manoeuvre, if there is the correct amount of slack in the lead, there will be a slight curve in its right atrial portion (Figure 15.1E). For lead stability the electrode must be securely sutured to the skin at its point of entry.

The pacing threshold usually rises to 2–3 V during the first few days after electrode insertion. The threshold should be checked daily and the voltage set at twice the measured threshold. Battery function and electrical connections should also be checked daily.

Pacing complications

Causes of failure to pace (Figure 15.3) include electrode displacement, myocardial perforation, exit block and a break in either the electrical connections or the pacing electrode.

Electrode displacement may cause intermittent or complete failure to pace. The electrode may fall back into the right atrial cavity and lead to atrial rather than ventricular pacing (Figure 15.4).

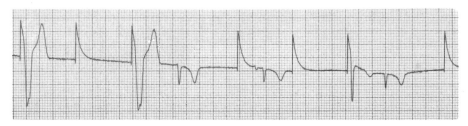

Figure 15.3 Intermittent failure to pace (lead II). Only the first and third pacing stimuli capture the ventricles

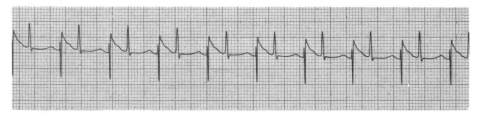

Figure 15.4 Atrial pacing. At the time of this recording, AV function was satisfactory so each pacing stimulus was followed by a narrow QRS complex after a PR interval of 0·22 s

Occasionally the electrode tip may perforate the thin right ventricular myocardium. This is more common with disposable electrodes, which tend to be stiffer than reusable ones. Failure to pace, diaphragmatic stimulation, pericardial friction rub and pericardial pain may result. Cardiac tamponade is extremely rare.

Sometimes pacing failure occurs without obvious electrode tip displacement or other cause. In these cases failure is attributed to 'exit block', the cause of which is thought to be excessive tissue reaction at the junction between electrode tip and endocardium.

A break in the electrical connection or in the electrode itself can be the cause of intermittent or complete pacing failure. In contrast to exit block, no pacing stimuli will appear on the ECG. Another occasional cause of pacing failure associated with absent pacing stimuli is external inhibition of a demand pacemaker usually resulting from electromagnetic waves being emitted from electrical equipment. This problem can be quickly solved by changing the pacemaker to fixed rate mode.

Pacemakers are most often used in the 'demand' mode, whereby the pacemaker senses spontaneous ventricular activity and only discharges a stimulus if a spontaneous beat has not occurred within a pre-set period. In some patients, particularly those with myocardial infarction, the signal generated by spontaneous activity may be too small for the pacemaker to sense. As a result, the pacemaker will function in a 'fixed rate' mode and pacing stimuli will be discharged at inappropriate times, and may fall on the T wave of a spontaneous beat (Figure 15.5). This is particularly undesirable in acute myocardial infarction because of the risk of precipitating ventricular fibrillation.

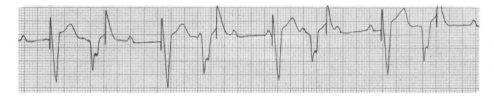

Figure 15.5 Failure to sense in a demand ventricular pacemaker. The first, third, fifth and seventh pacing stimuli capture the ventricles. The second, fourth, sixth and eighth stimuli fall on the T waves of spontaneous ventricular beats

As an alternative to electrode repositioning, unipolar pacing can be adopted. In contrast to bipolar pacing, the anode is remote from the electrode tip. The signal generated by spontaneous activity sensed between two poles separated by a large distance is much greater. Unipolar pacing can be achieved by disconnecting the pacemaker connection to the proximal pole of the pacing electrode and connecting it to a needle inserted beneath the skin in a convenient position which functions as the remote pole.

The site of entry of a transvenous pacing electrode can become infected: sometimes bacteraemia results. Infection will not clear up without removal of the pacing electrode. If necessary, a new pacing electrode will have to be inserted at a different site.

AV sequential pacing

Ventricular pacing results in dissociation between atrial and ventricular activity. When ventricular systole is not immediately preceded by atrial systole, cardiac output falls by up to one-third. Both the atria and ventricles may be paced sequentially so that the normal sequence of cardiac chamber activation can be maintained (Figure 15.6). In patients with a low cardiac output, AV sequential pacing can produce an important improvement in cardiac function.

Usually, AV sequential pacing is achieved by passing two leads to the heart: one to the atria and one to the ventricles. The best method of ensuring that an atrial lead is not displaced is to use one with a pre-formed J-shaped terminal portion. A

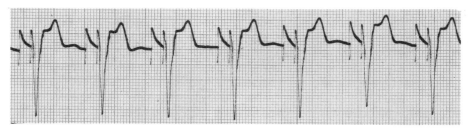

Figure 15.6 AV sequential pacing. Pacing stimuli precede both atrial and ventricular complexes

lead of this type can easily be positioned in the right atrial appendage (see Chapter 16). Recently, 'single-pass' leads with a distal electrode for ventricular pacing and a proximal pole for atrial pacing have been introduced for AV sequential pacing.

Temporary transcutaneous and oesophageal pacing

Transcutaneous cardiac pacing was first attempted many years ago but was usually unsuccessful and caused severe discomfort due to skeletal muscle stimulation. Recently, considerable success with less discomfort has been achieved by using large surface area skin electrodes and stimuli of much longer duration than are used for endocardial stimulation (20–40 ms). The latest generation of transcutaneous pacemakers function in the demand mode and have a maximum output in the region of 150 mA. One electrode is applied to the front of the chest and the other to the back over the right scapula. Pacing is likely to stimulate the atria at the same time as the ventricles. It is not always possible to ascertain from the ECG that the heart is being stimulated: monitoring of an arterial pulse may be necessary.

With oesophageal pacing, a long impulse duration is necessary (10 ms). Success is more often encountered when stimulating the atria than the ventricles.

As with transvenous pacing, transcutaneous and oesophageal pacing is unlikely to be successful after a prolonged period of cardiac arrest.

Main points

◆ Indications for temporary transvenous pacing include bifascicular, second- and third-degree AV block due to acute anterior infarction; 'complicated' second- and third-degree AV block due to acute inferior infarction; and recent syncope or near-syncope due to chronic disease of the sinus node or AV junction while awaiting implantation of a long-term pacemaker.

◆ Subclavian vein puncture is usually the best method of venous access for temporary pacing.

◆ The pacemaker stimulation threshold, battery function and electrical connections should be checked daily.

◆ AV sequential pacing improves cardiac output as compared with ventricular pacing and should be considered in those patients whose haemodynamic status is not satisfactory with ventricular pacing.

Chapter 16

Long-term cardiac pacing for bradycardias

This subject is discussed in detail to provide a concise account of the practical aspects of pacemaker implantation and the care of patients with pacemakers; often the remit of a cardiac department's junior members.

An artificial cardiac pacemaker generates electrical stimuli which can initiate myocardial contraction. The stimuli are usually delivered to the heart by transvenous leads or less commonly via epicardial, oesophageal or transthoracic electrodes.

The first pacemaker was implanted in 1958. Over the following 25 years, rapid progress in technology and an increasing awareness of the benefits of pacing have led to pacemakers being widely used. Patients of all ages, from the newborn to over 100 years old, have been paced: the average age at first implantation is 72 years.

In the United Kingdom, surveys have suggested that the annual rate of new pacemaker implantation should be in the order of 200 patients per million of the population. The implantation rate has increased over the years and is approaching this figure though there are some health districts that continue to have very low implantation rates. In 1986 implantation rates for USA, France, Belgium, and Germany were much higher than those in the United Kingdom: approximately 400 per million per year.

Indications for long-term cardiac pacing

The main considerations in deciding whether to implant a pacemaker are whether relief of symptoms and/or improvement in prognosis will be achieved. In some patients with asymptomatic impairment of the specialized cardiac conducting system, other factors may also be pertinent such as the need for medication which may cause unwanted bradycardia, or concern in a motor vehicle driver that an accident might result should syncope occur.

Clearly, long-term pacing is not indicated if bradycardia is unlikely to recur, e.g. if caused by drug toxicity or acute myocardial ischaemia.

Complete atrioventicular block

The most common reason for pacemaker implantation is prevention of syncope or near-syncope caused by complete AV block. A single episode is a sufficient indication and since the next blackout may cause injury or be fatal, delay should be minimal. Even in patients with a short life expectancy, pacing should be considered if by preventing syncope, independence may be preserved and serious injury, which may lead to greater demands on medical resources than pacing, may be avoided.

Complete heart block can reduce cardiac output and thereby lead to exertional dyspnoea and sometimes to cardiac failure. Pacing usually but not invariably improves these problems. Mental impairment is sometimes attributed to heart block but does not always improve with pacing: if there is doubt, it is best to undertake a trial of temporary pacing.

Without pacing, the prognosis in patients with complete heart block is poor. With an artificial pacemaker, life expectancy closely approaches that of the general population though those with overt coronary heart disease or with heart failure have a less good outlook. Pacemaker implantation should be considered in asymptomatic patients with complete AV block, particularly when the ventricular rate is 40 beats per minute or less, on purely prognostic grounds.

Narrow ventricular complexes during complete AV block suggests that interruption in conduction is at AV nodal level and that, in contrast to infranodal block, a subsidiary pacemaker within the His bundle will discharge reliably at a relatively rapid ventricular rate. However, in practice patients with narrow ventricular complexes during complete heart block may experience syncope and impaired exercise tolerance. In the United Kingdom, one-third of patients who receive pacemakers for complete AV block have narrow QRS complexes.

Congenital heart block
Congenital heart block, i.e. complete AV block that is discovered as a neonate or child and is not caused by acquired disease, is widely regarded as benign. However, some patients do develop symptoms or die suddenly. In asymptomatic patients the risks of not implanting a pacemaker have to be weighed against the possibility of complications associated with several decades of pacing. Unpaced patients should undergo ambulatory and exercise electrocardiography at regular intervals.

Second-degree AV block

The approach to second-degree AV block is similar to that for complete AV block. Mobitz II AV block often progresses to complete AV block. A recent study showed that symptoms were commonly associated with Mobitz II AV block and that whereas the prognosis was poor in unpaced patients it was similar to that of the general population in paced patients. This study also refuted the previously held view that Mobitz I AV block is benign in that the incidence of symptoms, prognosis and influence of pacing were the same as for patients with Mobitz II block. This poor outlook does not, however, apply to young people with transient and often nocturnal Wenkebach block which is due to high vagal tone and is benign.

First-degree AV block

First-degree AV block is not itself an indication for cardiac pacing. If a patient presents with first-degree block and syncope or near-syncope it is quite possible that the symptoms are due to transient second- or third-degree AV block but a pacemaker should not be implanted without proof of this, e.g. by ambulatory electrocardiography.

Bundle branch and fascicular blocks

The risk of high-degree AV block developing in an asymptomatic patient with either left or right bundle branch block is extremely small, and pacing is not indicated. In patients who present with syncope or near-syncope the approach should be the same as for first-degree AV block.

In bifascicular block the remaining functioning fascicle may fail to conduct, intermittently or persistently, and cause high-degree AV block. In patients with a good history of Adams–Stokes attacks, pacemaker implantation is indicated to prevent syncope without further investigation. With atypical symptoms, high-degree AV block must be documented first.

In asymptomatic bifascicular block, the chances of progression to complete AV block is in the order of 2% per year and the major determinants of prognosis are the presence of coronary artery or myocardial disease: prophylactic pacing is generally not indicated. Additional first-degree AV block or His bundle electrographic evidence of prolonged infranodal conduction suggest that conduction in the functioning fascicle is also impaired. However, there is no evidence of a higher risk.

AV and bundle branch block after myocardial infarction

AV block due to inferior myocardial infarction usually resolves within a few days and almost always by 3 weeks. When anterior infarction is complicated by high-degree AV block, there is usually extensive myocardial damage and hence the prognosis is poor: though block may persist it is prudent to ensure that the patient is going to survive before implanting a pacemaker. Thus pacemaker implantation should not be considered unless second- or third-degree AV block is present 3 weeks after myocardial infarction.

When a patient is admitted to hospital with heart block, there is often an unnecessary delay before referral for long-term pacing while myocardial infarction is excluded. Unless the patient has experienced typical cardiac pain or there are obvious ECG changes of recent infarction, AV block has probably not been caused by acute infarction.

Bifascicular block persisting after acute anterior infarction complicated by AV block raises the possibility that complete AV block might recur. Intermittent heart block has been demonstrated to occur in some patients with post-infarction bifascicular block and may necessitate pacing. However, prophylactic pacing does not reduce mortality.

Sick sinus syndrome

Sick sinus syndrome accounts for one-quarter of pacemaker implantations. Pacing is indicated when syncope or near-syncope are caused. Sinus bradycardia and pauses in sinus node activity for up to 2·0 s, particularly if nocturnal, can be physiological.

In patients with the bradycardia–tachycardia syndrome, pacing may be required to avoid severe bradycardia caused by anti-arrhythmic drugs. Sometimes tachyarrhythmias which start during bradycardia will be prevented by atrial pacing.

Pacing for sick sinus syndrome does not improve prognosis and is not usually indicated in asymptomatic patients. However, pauses in cardiac activity for several seconds might be considered an indication for pacing in those who operate machinery, including a motor car, to avoid an accident should syncope occur.

Hypersensitive carotid sinus syndrome

This term refers to patients who suffer from near-syncope or syncope without evidence of impaired function of the sinus node or AV junction in whom unilateral carotid sinus massage for 5 s causes sinus arrest or complete AV block for at least 3 s: pacing is indicated. Pacing is not indicated in asymptomatic patients with hypersensitive carotid sinus reflexes.

Pacing modes

The first generation of pacemakers functioned in a fixed-rate mode: the pacemaker stimulated the ventricles regularly, usually at 70 beats per minute, irrespective of any spontaneous cardiac activity (Figure 16.1). Competition with a spontaneous rhythm could cause irregular palpitation (Figure 16.2), and stimulation during ventricular repolarization could initiate ventricular fibrillation.

Subsequent developments enabled sensing of spontaneous activity via the stimulating lead to facilitate demand pacing: a sensed event resets the timing of delivery of the next pacemaker stimulus to avoid competition with spontaneous activity (Figure 16.3).

With the advent of reliable transvenous atrial pacing leads it became straightforward

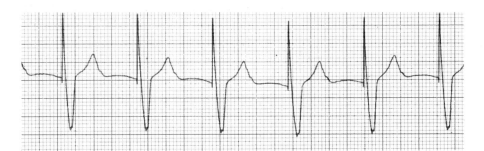

Figure 16.1 Fixed rate ventricular pacing at 71 beats/min

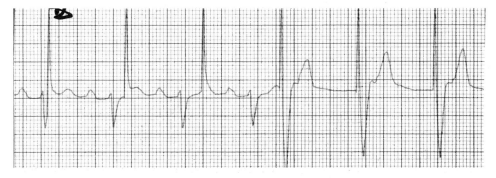

Figure 16.2 Fixed rate ventricular pacing in a patient with first-degree AV block. The first three stimuli fall during the refractory period and are ineffective. The fourth causes a premature contraction

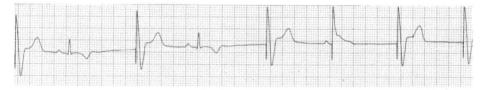

Figure 16.3 Demand ventricular pacemaker. The pacemaker is inhibited by the sinus beats (second and fourth complexes). The sixth complex is a fusion beat. A 'P' wave can be seen to precede the pacing stimulus. By chance, a sinus impulse has arisen at the instant when the pacemaker was set to discharge, and the ventricles have been activated by both stimulus impulse and pacemaker. Fusion beats should not be confused with failure to pace

to pace and sense in the atrium as well as the ventricle thus allowing both atrial and ventricular 'single chamber' pacing and also 'dual chamber' pacing whereby stimulation and/or sensing can take place at both atrial and ventricular levels. These developments have permitted a more physiological approach to cardiac stimulation.

Pacing system code

A five letter code is widely used to describe the various pacing modes; the first three characters are the most important.

The first character identifies the chamber or chambers that are paced: 'A' for atrium, 'V' for ventricle and 'D' (for double) if both atrium and ventricle can be stimulated.

The second character indicates the chamber or chambers whose activity is sensed: in addition to the use of 'A', 'V' and 'D', 'O' indicates that the pacemaker is insensitive.

The third character denotes the response to the sensed information: 'I' indicates that pacemaker output is inhibited by a sensed event, 'T' that stimulation is triggered by a sensed event and 'D' that ventricular sensed events inhibit pacemaker output while atrial sensed events trigger ventricular stimulation: 'O' indicates that there is no response to sensed events.

The fourth character denotes whether the generator is programmable. 'O' indicates that it is not; 'P' that it is a simple programmable unit (for one of two parameters, e.g. rate and output) and 'M' that it is multiprogrammable. 'C' indicates that, in addition, the pacemaker has facilities for telemetry. The facility for rate modulation in response to a sensed variable (see below) is denoted by 'R'.

The fifth character relates to antitachycardia functions: 'O', none; 'P', antitachycardia pacing (low energy stimulation); 'S', shock (i.e. cardioversion or defibrillation); and 'D', both antitachycardia pacing and shock.

Single chamber pacing

Ventricular demand pacing
In the absence of spontaneous ventricular activity, a ventricular demand pacemaker, like a fixed-rate unit, delivers stimuli to the ventricles at a regular rate. However, if spontaneous activity is sensed via the ventricular lead, the timing of delivery of the next pacemaker output is reset to avoid competition.

In ventricular inhibited (VVI) pacemakers a sensed event terminates the current stimulation cycle, thus inhibiting pacemaker output, and starts a new cycle (Figure 16.3). In contrast, a sensed event during the less commonly used mode of ventricular

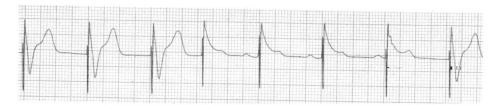

Figure 16.4 Ventricular triggered pacemaker. After the first three paced beats there is sinus rhythm. A pacing stimulus is discharged immediately after the onset of the QRS complex in these beats

triggered (VVT) pacing immediately triggers delivery of a pacing stimulus which will consequently fall during the myocardial refractory period and will thus be ineffective: the subsequent cycle will then start from delivery of the triggered impulsive (Figure 16.4).

The pacemaker is rendered insensitive immediately after a paced or sensed event for an interval which approximates the duration of myocardial depolarization and repolarization to prevent sensing the ventricular electrogram which is produced by the event; this interval (250–300 ms) is referred to as the refractory period.

Ventricular demand pacing is the most commonly employed mode but its use is diminishing as its disadvantages – the inabilities to facilitate the normal sequence of cardiac chamber activation and to provide a chronotropic response to exercise – become more widely appreciated (see below).

Unequivocal indications for ventricular demand pacing include bradycardia associated with persistent atrial fibrillation, second- and third-degree AV block in patients who are limited by impaired cerebral or locomotor function and patients with infrequent bradycardia in whom the pacemaker is mainly on 'stand-by'.

Atrial demand pacing
The timing cycles of atrial inhibited (AAI) and the less commonly used atrial triggered (AAT) modes are the same as for ventricular demand pacing, as described above (Figure 16.5). With atrial pacing, the refractory period is usually longer to avoid sensing the 'far field' ventricular electrogram which may be sensed via the atrial lead and which may inappropriately inhibit the pacemaker.

Atrial pacing is indicated for treatment of the sick sinus syndrome unless AV conduction is impaired. By stimulating the atria rather than the ventricles, the normal sequence of cardiac chamber activation is maintained, loss of which can reduce cardiac output by up to one-third. Sick sinus syndrome can be associated with impaired AV

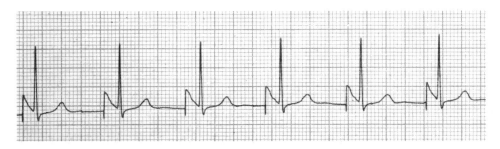

Figure 16.5 Atrial pacing

conduction. However, if there was no evidence of it at the time of pacemaker implantation the development of impaired AV conduction is uncommon. If atrial pacing at a rate of 120 beats/min causes second-degree AV block, AV conduction is probably impaired and dual chamber pacing would be indicated.

Dual chamber pacing

AV sequential pacing

In AV sequential (DVI) pacing the atria are stimulated first and then, after a delay which approximates the normal PR interval, the ventricles are stimulated (Figure 16.6). The pacemaker is inhibited by spontaneous ventricular activity but no sensing occurs in the atrium. As with other dual chamber modes, both atrial and ventricular electrodes are required.

There are non-commited and committed versions of AV sequential pacing. With the former, a sensed ventricular event during the interval between atrial and ventricular stimulation will inhibit delivery of the ventricular stimulus. With the latter, ventricular stimulation will always follow the atrial stimulus.

Fusion beats (Figure 16.7) are commonly seen during DVI pacing and are sometimes misinterpreted as pacemaker malfunction: whereas the pacemaker is inhibited by an event sensed in the ventricles, the first chamber to be stimulated is the atrium. Pacemaker output may therefore occur at the same time as spontaneous atrial activation because its resultant ventricular depolarization has not yet occurred.

Recently, the mode of DDI pacing has been introduced. Sensing occurs at atrial as well as ventricular levels but unlike DDD pacing (see below) sensed atrial events do not trigger ventricular stimulation. Thus this mode cannot facilitate endless loop tachycardia, a complication of dual chamber pacing which is described below.

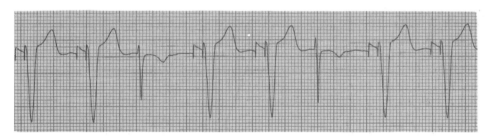

Figure 16.6 AV sequential pacing. Pacing stimuli precede both atrial and ventricular complexes. Pacing is inhibited by two spontaneous ventricular beats (DVI pacing)

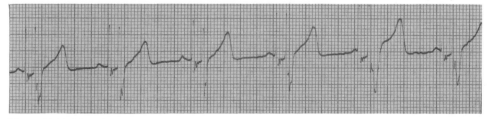

Figure 16.7 DVI pacing: fusion beats

The main indications for AV sequential pacing are sick sinus syndrome associated with impaired AV conduction and carotid sinus syndrome.

Atrial synchronized ventricular pacing
In this mode, ventricular stimulation is triggered by a sensed atrial event after an interval similar to the normal PR interval (Figure 16.8). It thereby maintains the normal sequence of cardiac chamber activation and permits a chronotropic response to exercise provided sinus node function is normal.

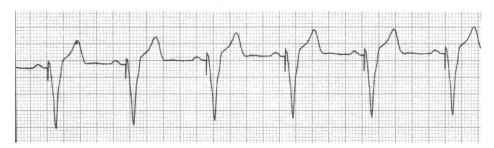

Figure 16.8 Atrial synchronized pacing. Each P wave is followed by a paced ventricular beat

If an atrial event is not sensed, ventricular stimulation continues at a fixed and usually fairly long cycle length – otherwise atrial standstill might lead to ventricular asystole. To avoid atrial tachycardia or fibrillation triggering inappropriately fast ventricular pacing rates, there is an atrial refractory interval: the atrial channel is rendered insensitive during the AV delay and for a period after ventricular stimulation. Sensed atrial activity at a cycle length shorter than this period will not trigger ventricular stimulation. The upper rate at which atrial activity will trigger ventricular output is determined by the 'total atrial refractory period' which consists of the AV delay plus the post-ventricular stimulus refractory period. For example, if the AV delay is 125 ms and the atrial refractory period is 250 ms, the upper rate limit will be $60\,000/375 = 160$ beats/min.

In earlier years, sensing only took place in the atrium and pacing only occurred in the ventricle (VAT). Thus ventricular ectopic beats or rhythms faster than the sinus node rate would not inhibit ventricular output. Subsequently, VDD pacing was introduced whereby sensing takes place in the ventricles as well so that spontaneous ventricular activity will inhibit the pacemaker (Figure 16.9).

Atrial synchronized ventricular pacing is indicated in second- and third-degree AV block when sinus node function is normal. It is contraindicated in sick sinus syndrome or when there are atrial tachyarrhythmias.

'Endless loop tachycardia'
If a ventricular stimulus is conducted retrogradely to the atria via either the AV junction or, if present, an accessory AV pathway, and the timing of the resultant atrial activation is outside the pacemaker's atrial refractory period, it will trigger ventricular stimulation and hence initiate an 'endless loop tachycardia' (Figure 16.10). The tachycardia is also referred to as 'pacemaker mediated tachycardia'. Ventriculo-atrial conduction has been demonstrated in approximately two-thirds of patients

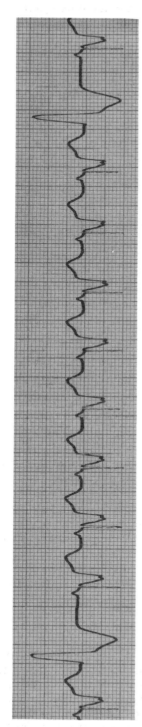

Figure 16.9 VDD pacing, demonstrating chronotropic response to exercise and inhibition by ventricular ectopic beats

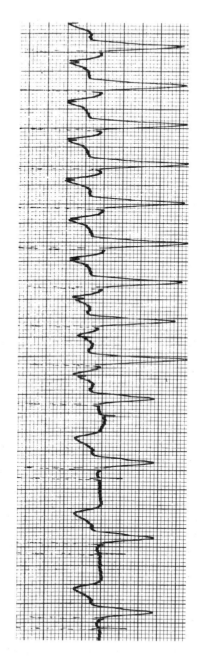

Figure 16.10 Pacemaker-mediated tachycardia develops after four cycles of AV sequential pacing

with sick sinus syndrome and one-fifth of those with complete AV block. Endless loop tachycardia can usually be prevented by prolongation of the atrial refractory period but at the expense of reduction of the upper rate limit for ventricular stimulation. Endless loop tachycardia can be avoided in 90% of patients by setting the AV delay to 125 ms and the post-ventricular atrial refractory period to 300 ms.

Pacemakers are now available that can detect endless loop tachycardia and interrupt it by prolonging the atrial refractory period for one cycle.

AV universal pacing
In this mode (DDD), both sensing and pacing can take place at atrial and ventricular levels. Universal pacing allows the pacemaker to function in atrial demand (AAI), AV sequential (DVI) or atrial synchronized (VDD) modes depending on the spontaneous heart rhythm (Figure 16.11). If there is sinus bradycardia it functions as an atrial demand pacemaker. If there is impaired AV conduction, ventricular pacing is triggered by either spontaneous atrial activity or by delivery of an atrial stimulus. When sinus node function is normal, it functions in the atrial synchronized mode thus providing a chronotropic response to exercise. The pacemaker is inhibited by both atrial and ventricular ectopic beats. Endless loop tachycardia may occur if there is retrograde AV conduction.

DDD pacing is indicated in second- and third-degree AV block and in sinus node dysfunction. Atrial tachyarrhythmias are a contraindication.

'Physiological pacing'

Ventricular demand pacing presents the least technical challenge and continues to be the most commonly employed pacing mode. However, the inabilities to maintain the normal sequence of cardiac chamber activation and to provide a chronotropic response to exercise are important disadvantages.

Atrial synchronized ventricular pacing
This mode which both maintains AV synchronization and facilitates a chronotropic response has been shown to increase cardiac output at rest and during exercise as compared with ventricular pacing at 70 beats/min. Exercise capacity has been measured on a double-blind basis during ventricular pacing at 70 beats/min and during atrial synchronized ventricular pacing. The latter mode has been shown to increase maximal exercise capacity by approximately 30%. However, individual patients varied in the degree by which they benefited: in a few there was little improvement whereas in a significant proportion there was a dramatic increase. Neither age nor cause of heart block predicted the amount of benefit. It used to be thought that 'physiological' pacing was of greatest value to patients with poor ventricular function. This is not the case; indeed, patients with high venous pressures may not benefit.

Atrial synchronized pacing improves parameters in addition to maximal exercise tolerance. Shortness of breadth, dizziness and palpitation are less frequent whereas fixed rate pacing tends to impair the normal blood pressure response to exercise and leads to a higher respiratory rate and perceived exertion during submaximal exercise. The advantages of atrial synchronized pacing have been shown to be maintained long term.

There are limitations to atrial synchronized ventricular pacing. First, normal or at least near-normal sinus node activity is required. Secondly, the current generation

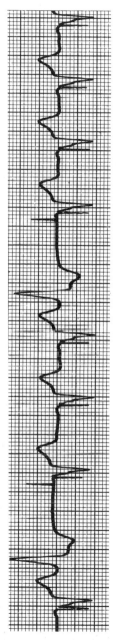

Figure 16.11 Universal (DDD) pacing. Spontaneous P waves can be seen to trigger ventricular stimulation. After the first and fifth paced beats there are ventricular ectopic beats which inhibit the pacemaker. There is sinus node depression following the extrasystoles to which the pacemaker responds by pacing the atria as well as the ventricles

of pacemakers cannot distinguish between a rise in atrial rate caused by a physiological increase in sinus node activity and that due to an atrial tachyarrhythmia. Thirdly, an atrial as well as a ventricular pacing lead is required.

Rate response systems
In terms of exercise capacity, the ability to increase heart rate is far more important than maintaining atrioventricular synchronization. This has been demonstrated by measuring exercise tolerance during three pacing modes: fixed rate, atrial synchronized and ventricular pacing at a rate commensurate with but not synchronized to atrial activity. Both the latter forms of chronotropic pacing increased exercise performance to a similar degree as compared with fixed rate pacing.

   Several pacing systems are available or are being developed that can facilitate a chronotropic response independent of atrial activity: a change in stimulation rate is achieved in response to a parameter that alters with exercise. These have the advantages of requiring only one pacing lead, of not necessitating normal sinus node activity and of not causing endless loop tachycardia.

Evoked QT response
Though it has been known for many years that the QT interval decreases with increasing heart rate, it has only recently been appreciated that sympathetic nervous system activity is a major independent determinant of QT interval duration: QT interval shortens during exercise even during fixed rate pacing. The pacemaker senses, via a conventional ventricular pacing electrode, the interval between pacing stimulus and apex of the evoked T wave: a decrease in the interval leads to an increase in stimulation rate.

Muscle vibration
A system that senses vibration resulting from muscle activity using a piezo-electric crystal attached to the inner surface of the pacemaker provides a satisfactory chronotropic response to exercise. It can be used for atrial as well as ventricular pacing.

Respiratory rate
There is a close relation between respiratory and heart rates. An implantable system is available whose discharge rate is governed by the respiratory rate which is monitored by means of an electrode implanted subcutaneously in the chest wall, using the impedance principle. A system using changes in intravascular impedance monitored by a conventional bipolar lead as a measure of respiration has also been developed.

Blood temperature
Skeletal muscle activity generates heat which is transferred to the blood. There is a useful relation between level of exercise and right ventricular blood temperature. One problem, however, is that there is a latency in the system due to the delay of 1 or 2 minutes before blood temperature rises after the start of exercise.

Other sensors
Blood pH, P_{CO_2}, P_{O_2}, the integral of the intracardiac ventricular complex and right ventricular stroke volume are other parameters that are being investigated for use in rate responsive pacing. Information on long-term reliability of sensors is not yet available. Rate response systems that can use a conventional lead have practical advantages over systems that require a lead incorporating a specialized sensor.

'Multisensor pacing'
Dual chamber pacemakers are now available which in addition to sensing atrial activity will respond to parameters related to exercise such as vibration or QT interval.

'Pacemaker syndrome'
It is at rest that the disadvantage of loss of AV synchrony caused by ventricular pacing may become apparent. When normal AV synchronization is lost, atrial contraction may occur against closed mitral and tricuspid valves. Atrial pressure will rise and impede venous return so that during the next diastolic period the ventricles will be underfilled with resultant reduction in stroke volume. Loss of properly timed atrial systole results in a reduction in cardiac output of up to one-third and hence a fall in blood pressure (Figure 16.12) which may cause hypotension: near-syncope and syncope can result. Ventriculoatrial conduction (Figure 16.13) causes even greater haemodynamic upset: the resultant atrial distension may actually initiate a reflex vasodepressor effect.

Hypotension is likely to be more marked whilst standing. It is most severe during the first few seconds of ventricular pacing, before vasoconstrictor compensatory mechanisms can come into play, so ventricular pacing is particularly unsuitable for patients who are mainly in sinus rhythm but who often develop bradycardia at a rate less than the cycle length of the ventricular pacemaker, i.e. those with sick sinus or carotid sinus syndromes. Atrioventricular sequential pacing or, when AV conduction is not impaired, atrial pacing will avoid this problem. This has been demonstrated by recording ambulatory blood pressure in patients with ventricular demand pacemakers. The onset of ventricular pacing was followed by hypotension which was greater in those who had complained of syncope and near-syncope. AV sequential pacing prevented hypotension and syncope.

Pacemaker hardware

Pulse generator
A pulse generator consists of a power source together with electronic circuits to control the timing and characteristics of the impulses that it generates.

In the past, several power sources have been used including mercury–zinc cells, rechargeable nickel–cadmium cells and nuclear energy. Now, lithium iodide cells are used almost exclusively. They have replaced the other widely used power source, the mercury–zinc cell, whose lifetime was limited to 24–48 months and which produced hydrogen making it impractical to hermetically seal the pacemaker. Lithium pacemakers have a lifespan of 4–15 years and a predictable, progressive discharge behaviour. They are contained in a hermetically sealed titanium can, weigh 35–50 g, and generally have a maximum diameter of no more than 50 mm and a thickness of as little as 6 mm.

Pacemaker leads
Stimuli produced by the pulse generator are conducted to the heart via a lead which consists of an insulated wire with an electrode at its tip which is attached to the heart.

Leads that are sewn on to the epicardium or screwed into the myocardium necessitate thoracotomy and are now, with the advent of reliable transvenous leads, rarely used unless pacemaker implantation is undertaken at the time of open heart surgery, or venous thrombosis or tricuspid valve prosthesis preclude a transvenous approach.

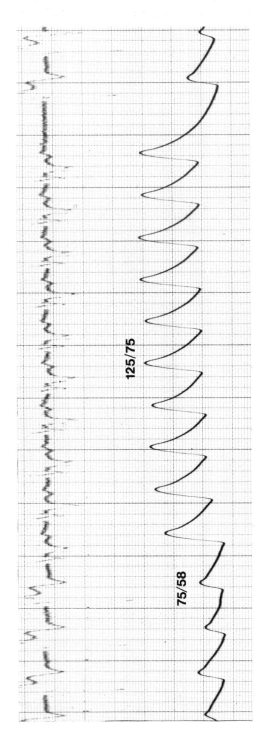

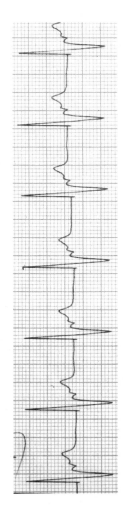

Figure 16.12 Pacemaker syndrome. Effect of ventricular pacing on arterial pressure. There was symptomatic hypotension during the right ventricular pacing. After the first four paced beats the pacemaker is inhibited by an external pacemaker (chest wall stimulation), allowing sinus rhythm to resume control of the heart with consequent increase in pressure. The arterial pressure falls during the last two beats, when ventricular pacing restarts

Figure 16.13 Ventricular pacing with retrograde activation (lead II). Each ventricular complex is followed by a P wave

Transvenous leads are used in over 95% of pacemaker implantations. A modern lead consists of a multifilar, helically coiled wire which is insulated by a material that does not cause tissue reaction or thrombosis: silicone rubber or polyurethane.

At the lead tip is the cathode which is composed of an inert material such as platinum–iridium, eligiloy, steel or vitreous carbon. For effective stimulation, this must be securely and closely attached to the endocardium. If fibrous tissue, which is non-excitable, develops between cathode and endocardium the amount of energy required to stimulate the heart will increase and may exceed the output capability of the pacemaker.

To achieve a low threshold for stimulation and secure endocardial attachment, several 'fixation devices' have been employed. 'Passive' fixation devices include tines, flanges or fins positioned proximal to the lead tip which can become entrapped in the trabeculae. 'Active' devices include an electrode in the shape of a helix which by rotation of the lead can be wound around a trabeculum, and a retractable metal screw which can be screwed into the endo-myocardium. Recently, 'porous' metal or carbon electrodes have been introduced: the surface of the cathode consists of many microscopic pores which promote rapid tissue ingrowth and hence very secure fixation. Movement between electrode and endocardium and thus generation of fibrous tissue is minimized. One new electrode elutes dexamethasone to minimize local tissue reaction and hence stimulation threshold. Attachment of atrial leads was impracticable until the advent of fixation devices. The distal portion of atrial leads are often 'J' shaped to facilitate positioning in the right atrial appendage.

The amount of energy required to stimulate the heart is related to the surface area of the cathode. Nowadays, low surface area electrodes are used – 6–12 mm^2.

Unipolar versus bipolar pacing
In unipolar pacing the anode is remote from the heart, usually the metal can containing the pulse generator. In bipolar pacing, which is less widely used, both anode and cathode are within the cardiac chamber to be paced, the anode positioned along the lead near to its cathodal tip. A commonly held view is that an electrogram sensed by a unipolar lead is larger than that from a bipolar lead. There is in fact usually no difference between bipolar and unipolar electrograms or stimulation thresholds. Bipolar pacing has the advantage that inappropriate sensing of electromagnetic interference and skeletal muscle electromyograms is much less likely, as is extra-cardiac stimulation. Reasons for favouring unipolar pacing are that there is greater experience with unipolar leads, that leads have in the past been thinner and surface ECG unipolar pacemaker spikes are larger. Furthermore, until the recent introduction of 'in-line' connectors to the pulse generator it was necessary with bipolar pacing to utilize two bulky connectors.

Costs
In the United Kingdom, the current approximate costs of a pulse generator plus leads for single chamber, programmable single chamber and dual chambered pacing systems are £500, £850 and £1700, respectively.

Pacemaker implantation

Facilities for fluoroscopy, ECG monitoring and cardiopulmonary resuscitation are required. The procedure is usually carried out under local anaesthesia and takes 15–45 minutes.

Subclavian approach

The subclavian approach is now widely used and is especially useful if more than one lead is to be inserted. The pacemaker lead(s) are introduced via infraclavicular subclavian vein puncture and are connected to the pulse generator which is implanted in a subcutaneous pocket fashioned over pectoralis major.

An incision is made 2 cm below the junction of the middle and inner thirds of the clavicle and is extended in a lateral and usually inferior direction for approximately 7 cm. A subcutaneous pocket large enough to accommodate the pulse generator is created by blunt dissection.

Puncture of the subclavian vein is easier if the vein is distended: a slight head-down position will help. A needle is introduced just below the inferior border of the clavicle at the junction of its middle and inner thirds and directed towards the sternoclavicular joint so that it passes behind the posterior surface of the clavicle. As the needle punctures the vein, venous blood will be aspirated easily: only a trickle suggests that the needle is not in the vein. Aspiration of air or bright pulsatile blood indicate puncture of the pleura or subclavian artery, respectively. If the patient has a 'deep' chest, and particularly if the clavicle bows anteriorly, it may be necessary to introduce the needle a little more laterally and to point it slightly posteriorly.

Cannulation of the vein is then achieved by introducing a flexible guide wire, preferably with a J-shaped tip, through the needle. Resistance to its passage indicates that the wire is not in the vein. The wire is passed into the superior vena cava and its position checked by fluoroscopy. The needle is then withdrawn and a sheath within which is a vessel dilator is passed over the wire into the vein. The guide wire and dilator are then removed and the pacing lead inserted into the sheath. If it is planned to introduce a second pacing lead, then the guide wire can be left in place to permit introduction of a second introducer and sheath. 'Peel-away' sheaths are used so that their removal is not prevented by the connector at the proximal end of the lead.

Cephalic vein approach

An alternative to subclavian vein puncture is to cut down onto the cephalic vein in the deltopectoral groove. This approach avoids the risks of subclavian vein puncture but has its own disadvantages. The vein may not be big enough to accommodate two leads and sometimes is even too small for one lead. It is sometimes difficult to manipulate the lead from the cephalic vein into the superior vena cava.

Occasionally, a cut-down technique is used with the jugular, axillary or pectoral veins.

Positioning of a ventricular lead

To facilitate manipulation of long-term pacing leads, which are very flexible, a wire stylet is passed down the centre of the lead. Bending the distal part of the stylet or its partial withdrawal will often aid positioning.

The lead is passed into the right atrium (see Figure 15.1). Sometimes the lead can then be directly advanced through the tricuspid valve to the right ventricular apex. More often, it is necessary to form a loop in the atrium by impinging the lead tip on the atrial wall and then advancing the lead a little further. By rotating the lead its tip can then be positioned near the tricuspid valve. Slight withdrawal of the lead will allow it to'flick' through the valve into the ventricle. Ventricular ectopic beats are usually provoked as the valve is crossed. If these do not occur then the coronary sinus may have been entered. Entry into the ventricle can be confirmed by advancing the lead into the pulmonary artery. Once in the right ventricle, the lead tip is positioned in or near the ventricular apex by a process of lead rotation, advancement and withdrawal. A stable position should be ensured by checking for continuous pacing and for absence of excessive lead tip movement during deep inspiration and coughing. Once a satisfactory position has been achieved both in terms of stability and measurements (see below), it is very important that the lead is secured by placing a short length of rubber sleeve around it near its point of entry into the vein and fixing it to the underlying muscle with a non-adsorbable suture.

Positioning of an atrial lead
The right atrial appendage is the usual site for atrial pacing. If necessary, atrial pacing may be performed from the coronary sinus or by using a 'screw-in' lead to pace from the septal or free right atrial walls.

For pacing the right atrial appendage, a lead with a J-shaped terminal portion is usually used. First, using a straight stylet the lead tip is straightened and advanced to the mid-right atrium. The lead is then rotated so that its tip is near the tricuspid valve. Partial withdrawal of the stylet causes the lead to assume its J shape and slight withdrawal of the lead itself allows the lead tip to enter the appendage. A straight lead may be positioned in the appendage by use of a stylet whose terminal 2–3 in have been shaped into a tight 'J'.

Correct positioning will be demonstrated by the lead tip moving from side to side with atrial systole. Lateral screening should demonstrate that the lead is pointing anteriorly. Lead stability should be confirmed by twisting the lead 45° in either direction: the lead tip should not turn. It is important that there is the correct amount of slack in the lead: during inspiration the angle between the two limbs of the J should not exceed 80°.

Measurement of stimulation and sensing thresholds
Achievement of low stimulation and sensing thresholds is essential for satisfactory long-term pacing. High thresholds suggest that the cathode is not in close apposition to excitable tissue. Thresholds rise after pacemaker implantation, usually peaking 3 weeks to 3 months after surgery. If they become high they may exceed the stimulation and sensing capabilities of the pulse generator.

Thresholds are usually measured with a commercially produced pacing systems analyser. It is preferable to match the analyser with the generator to be implanted so that they have similar impulse generating and sensing circuits. The same unipolar or bipolar electrode configuration should be used as is planned to use with the implanted system.

Stimulation threshold
The stimulation threshold is the smallest electrical stimulus (delivered by the cathode outside the ventricular effective and relative refractory periods) which will consistently depolarize the myocardium and thereby pace the heart.

To measure the stimulation threshold, the analyser is set to deliver impulses at 70 beats/min (or if there is no bradycardia at the time, 10 beats/min in excess of the spontaneous rate) with an impulse duration commensurate with that which the implanted pulse generator will deliver (often 0·5 ms) and a voltage output of 5 V. The threshold is then established by progressively reducing the output until failure of capture occurs: if the patient has no spontaneous rhythm, pacemaker output will have to be promptly increased to avoid asystole. At a pulse duration of 0·5 ms, a voltage threshold of less than 1·0 V is satisfactory: usually the threshold will be in the region of 0·5 V.

Strength–duration curve
The longer the duration of the pacing stimulus the more energy is delivered and hence the lower is the stimulation threshold. However, the relationship is not linear: the range of efficient impulse duration, in terms of energy consumption, is 0.25–1.0 ms. A strength–duration curve can be created by measuring the threshold, in terms of voltage, current (mA) or energy (μJ) at several different pulse durations. If the stimulation threshold is measured by progressively increasing the output from a subthreshold level it will be found to be slightly higher: the Wedensky phenomenon.

Sensing threshold
To ensure satisfactory sensing it is important to ensure the intracardiac electrogram resulting from spontaneous activity in the cardiac chamber to be paced is of sufficient amplitude. This is usually done using a pacing systems analyser. Ventricular and atrial electrograms should be greater than 4 mV and 2 mV, respectively. In 'borderline' cases the slew rate, i.e. the rate of change of signal voltage, is also important: low rates may result in failure to sense.

Lead impedance
The pacing systems analyser can also be used to measure lead impedance which is a measure of resistance to flow of current in the lead. It varies with lead type but is usually in the order of 400–800 Ω. A low impedance suggests a break in insulation and hence leakage of current whereas a high impedance points to lead fracture.

Complications of pacemaker implantation

Mild bruising is not uncommon but occasionally poor haemostasis will result in a haematoma which if tense should be evacuated.

Infection should occur in less than 1% of implantations and is virtually always staphyloccocal. Unless it is only superficial, explantation will usually be required even if antibiotics appear to help initially. It is usually not possible to remove a pacing lead safely with a fixation device without resorting to thoracotomy. The lead should be shortened so that it no longer lies in the infected area and its proximal end should be capped and fixed with a suture. Occasionally infection persists on the lead and causes a bacteraemia in which case thoracotomy may well be necessary.

Prophylactic antibiotics are widely used but there is no evidence that they are of value.

Erosion is a late complication but is often a consequence of implantation technique. Factors that predipose to erosion include creation of a pacemaker pocket which is too tight or too superficial, a very thin patient, and use of a generator with sharp corners. The skin will be found to be thinned around the site of erosion. Infection is often present but it is secondary to erosion. If 'threatened' erosion is detected the generator may be re-sited but if the skin is broken explantation will be necessary.

Lead displacement was once a common problem but with modern leads it occurs in less than 1% of implantations: it necessitates re-operation.

Complications of attempted subclavian vein puncture are infrequent: they include pneumothorax, haemothorax, air embolism, brachial plexus damage and puncture of the subclavian artery.

Fashioning of a generator pocket which is too large may allow spontaneous or intentional repeated rotation of the pulse generator which can cause dislodgement or fracture of the pacing lead: the 'twiddler's syndrome'.

Complications related to pulse generator

Electromyographic interference
This common problem is virtually confined to unipolar pacing systems. Myopotentials generated from the underlying muscle are sensed by the pacemaker as spontaneous cardiac activity (Figures 16.14 and 16.15). In systems where sensed events inhibits output, inappropriate cessation of pacing will occur. Short periods of electromyographic inhibition are common and usually asymptomatic. Longer periods may cause syncope and necessitate re-operation, or in programmable pacemakers (see below), adjustment to sensitivity, pacing mode or polarity.
   Susceptibility to electromyographic inhibition can be demonstrated by asking the patient to extend his arms and then press his hands firmly together. It is only significant if pacemaker inhibition lasts for several seconds, particularly if the patient's symptoms are reproduced.

Muscle stimulation
This complication is again related to unipolar pacing. It is a consequence of the pacemaker can being the anode: stimulation of the underlying pectoral muscle occurs and can be very troublesome. Most unipolar pacemakers now have an insulating covering applied to the back and sides of the pacemaker so that the only anodal contact is with the subcutaneous tissues.

Generator failure
Premature generator failure does occur occasionally, even at the time of implantation.

Complications related to pacing lead

Exit block
The development of excessive fibrous tissue, which is non-excitable, around the cathode may increase the stimulation threshold to a level higher than the pacemaker's output. The result will be intermittent or persistent failure to pace without evidence of lead displacement (see Figure 15.3). Exit block is most likely to occur in the first 3 weeks to 3 months after implantation when stimulation threshold is at its highest. Sometimes exit block is transient, otherwise lead repositioning will be required unless generator output can be increased by reprogramming (see below). Modern leads with low surface area, porous surfaced electrodes and positive fixation devices rarely give rise to this complication.

Lead fracture
With modern leads, fracture is rare. If it does occur it is usually at the point where the lead enters the venous system, at the site of a fixation suture or wherever there is excessive angulation of the lead. Lead fracture will cause intermittent or persistent failure to pace and sense. Lead fracture can often be detected radiographically but should not be confused with 'pseudofracture': the pressure of a tight ligature directly applied to the lead may compress the insulation and spread the coils of wire inside without interfering with lead function.

Insulation breakdown
This will allow leakage of current, which may cause stimulation of adjacent muscles, and hence premature battery depletion. A tight ligature anchoring the lead without use of a rubber sleeve is the commonest cause.

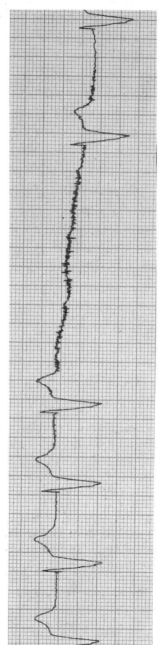

Figure 16.14 Electromyographic inhibition of a ventricular demand pacemaker. Each time the patient lifted his arm, he felt dizzy. Corrected by programming to VVT

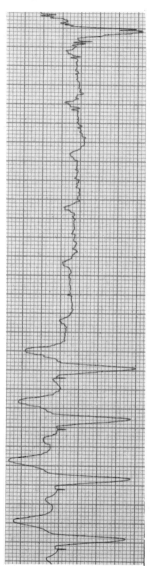

Figure 16.15 Electromyographic inhibition of a universal (DDD) pacemaker. Activities such as washing hands caused near-syncope. Corrected by decreasing pacemaker sensitivity

Phrenic nerve and diaphragmatic stimulation
The phrenic nerve or diaphragm can sometimes be stimulated through the intervening thin myocardial walls by atrial and ventricular leads respectively. Lead repositioning will be required unless, in programmable pacemakers, cessation of extra-cardiac stimulation can be achieved by output reduction.

Venous thrombosis
Clinically apparent subclavian vein thrombosis is rare and pulmonary embolism even rarer. Anticoagulant therapy is indicated. Angiographic studies have reported that asymptomatic venous thrombosis is not infrequent.

Pacemaker programmability

A programmable pacemaker can be non-invasively adjusted in one or more of its functions by radiofrequency signals emitted from an external programming device. Programmability enables achievement of optimal pacemaker function for the individual patient and can also be used in the diagnosis and treatment of certain pacemaker complications: it reduces the need for re-operation by one-fifth. Some authorities regard their use as mandatory.

Simple programmable pacemakers permit alteration to rate end output. In multiprogrammable pacemakers a wide variety of parameters can be adjusted. These are listed below together with typical options:

1. Lower rate limit (30–150 beats/min).
2. Output (2·5–5·0 V or 1–12 mA).
3. Sensitivity (0·5–8 mV).
4. Pacing mode (e.g. inhibited, triggered or fixed rate).
5. Refractory period (200–500 ms).
6. Pacing polarity (uni- or bipolar).
7. AV delay (0–250 ms) (for dual chamber pacemakers).
8. Upper rate limits (100–180 beats/min) (for dual chamber pacemakers).

Recently, software-based pacemakers have been introduced. Many functions are controlled by a microcomputer within the pacemaker which can be externally programmed: functions can be modified and new developments incorporated that had not even been anticipated at the time of implantation.

Some examples of the advantages of programmability are discussed below.

In patients who are mainly in sinus rhythm, reduction of the stand-by rate will allow sinus rhythm to be maintained for longer periods and will therefore help to avoid the haemodynamic disadvantages of ventricular pacing. Reduction of stimulation rate may occasionally help in the management of angina. Sometimes an increase in rate is helpful in the treatment of cardiac failure or arrhythmias.

Usually, the stimulation threshold is a lot lower than the maximum output of a pacemaker; a reduction in output will prolong battery life. At regular intervals, the threshold can be measured by progressive reduction in output and then the output programmed to the threshold value plus a safety margin. Extracardiac stimulation can often be stopped by reduction in output without approaching the threshold level. Some pacemakers have a high output facility (e.g. ability to increase output from 5 to 10 V): use of this may avoid the need for re-operation should exit block, which may be a temporary problem, occur.

Increase in sensitivity of the amplifier circuits may help with undersensing whereas inappropriate sensing of T waves or after-potentials may be dealt with by reduction in sensitivity or prolongation of refractory period.

Reduction in sensitivity may prevent electromyographic inhibition. Alternatively, reprogramming from inhibited to triggered mode will at least prevent bradycardia even if the electromyographic potentials reset the stimulation cycle. Another solution, which may also help with extra-cardiac stimulation, is to change from unipolar to bipolar pacing in systems that have this facility.

Atrial pacemakers require a higher sensitivity, because the atrial electrogram is usually of lower amplitude than its ventricular counterpart, and a longer refractory period to avoid sensing the far-field ventricular electrogram. A multiprogrammable generator can be adjusted for use as either an atrial or ventricular pacemaker.

In dual chamber pacing systems, prolongation of the atrial refractory period may prevent endless loop tachycardia. Sometimes endless loop tachycardia can be prevented by reducing sensitivity of the atrial channel so that the atrial electrogram during sinus rhythm is sensed but the atrial electrogram resulting from retrograde conduction, which is usually of lower amplitude, is not detected. In patients with sick sinus syndrome, reprogramming from DDD to DDI or DVI modes will prevent endless loop tachycardia. Alteration from DDD to VVI may be required should atrial fibrillation develop.

Pacemaker clinic

Patients with implanted pacemakers should regularly attend a follow-up clinic. The main purposes are to check that the pacemaker is working satisfactorily; to ensure that there are no pacing complications; to detect impending battery depletion so that generator replacement can be carried out before the patient is at risk; and to maintain a record of patients' locations should a recall of a particular generator or lead be necessary. Trans-telephonic ECG monitoring can be used to ensure satisfactory pacemaker function in between clinic visits.

The main indicator of impending battery depletion is a reduction in the stimulation rate which has to be measured precisely during fixed rate pacing usually initiated by placing a magnet over the pacemaker. Each type of pacemaker has its own characteristic 'end of life rate': it is usually in the order of a 5–10% reduction of the 'beginning of life' rate.

Some pulse generators have the facility to transmit data to the programmer, i.e. telemetry. Information about how the pacemaker has been programmed, battery status, stimulation and sensing thresholds, lead impedance, patient details and even intracardiac electrograms can be obtained. A rise in lead impedance suggests lead fracture.

Electromagnetic interference

External electromagnetic interference may be sensed by demand pacemakers and cause either inhibition or reversion to the fixed rate mode but the pacemaker will not be damaged. The many sources include electric motors in household devices, internal combustion engines, microwave ovens, radio transmitters, theft and weapon detection systems, arc welding apparatus and radar. In practice, however, very few problems are encountered and patients should be reassured that the risks are minimal. Clearly, if a patient feels dizzy near electrical equipment they should quickly walk away from it. If a patient's work brings him into close proximity with strong sources of electromagnetic interference a bipolar or triggered pacemaker should be implanted.

Cardioversion may cause pacemaker damage but this should be prevented if the paddles are at least 15 cm from the generator and preferably are positioned so they are at right angles to the pacing system. Pacemaker function should be checked after the procedure.

Diathermy may damage a pacemaker, cause inappropriate inhibition or possibly precipitate ventricular fibrillation. These risks can be avoided if the active electrode is kept at least 15 cm from the generator and the indifferent electrode sited as far away as possible so that its dipole is perpendicular to the pacing system. The pulse should be monitored so that diathermy could be interrupted if prolonged inhibition occurred.

Radiation for diagnostic purposes will not affect a pacemaker but therapeutic levels may cause damage. The pacemaker should be shielded, and if this is not possible re-siting of the generator should be considered.

Limited experience with magnetic resonance imaging indicates that all pacemakers will revert to fixed rate mode and some will pace at a dangerously fast rate.

Short-wave diathermy can cause pacemaker inhibition.

Advice on practical matters

Patients should be encouraged to lead a normal life. It may be prudent to avoid contact sports because of the risk of damage to the pacemaker or pacemaker site.

In the United Kingdom, the presence of complete heart block should be notified to the Licensing Centre and driving should not be permitted. Patients may resume driving 1 month after implantation of a pacemaker provided its function is checked regularly. However, patients are generally not allowed to hold a public or heavy goods vehicle licence, though exceptional cases may be considered by the Honorary Medical Advisory Panel.

There is no problems with air travel but patients should carry details about their pacemaker in case the pacemaker activates an airport metal detector and in case a pacing problem occurs while abroad.

A pacemaker must be explanted before cremation to avoid explosion.

Main points

- Long-term pacing is indicated in almost all cases of symptomatic bradycardia and should also be considered in asymptomatic patients with second- or third-degree AV block or long pauses in sinus node activity.

- Ventricular demand pacing prevents normal AV synchrony and does not permit a chronotropic response to exercise.

- Loss of AV synchrony may cause symptomatic hypotension (pacemaker syndrome) and can be prevented by atrial or AV sequential pacing.

- Absence of a chronotropic response to exercise can markedly reduce exercise tolerance. Atrial synchronized ventricular pacing and rate responsive systems sensitive to physiological parameters such as vibration, QT interval, respiration and blood temperature will facilitate a chronotropic response to exercise.

- The modern pacemaker is small, reliable and has a long battery life. Pacemaker infection is the commonest reason for re-operation. Many other complications can be resolved without operation if the pacemaker is programmable.

Chapter 17

Ambulatory ECG monitoring

Ambulatory ECG monitoring is an invaluable diagnostic tool. The technique consists of continuously recording the ECG, usually for a period of 24 hours, on magnetic tape using a portable battery operated tape recorder which is worn on a belt at the waist. If appropriate, the patient can be fully ambulant, carrying out his or her normal day-to-day activities.

The electrocardiogram is recorded by means of two electrodes applied to areas of thoroughly cleaned skin. Usually one electrode is placed over the manubrium sterni and the other electrode over the V5 chest lead position. As an alternative a modified V1 lead can be obtained by placing one electrode over the V1 chest lead position and the other electrode beneath the lateral part of the left clavicle. Some systems allow simultaneous recording of two leads. This increases diagnostic accuracy and aids in the detection of artefact which is unlikely to appear on both leads at the same time. Furthermore, sometimes one lead will not reveal important diagnostic information while another will (see Figures 2.4 and 6.22).

The tape recording is analysed in less than an hour by replaying it at 60–100 times real-time. Playback systems have facilities for printing out selected portions of the recording on ECG paper at standard speed. Most recording systems can automatically detect bradycardias, tachycardias and ectopic beats, though in practice an operator has to supervise the analysis.

Clinical applications

Only clinical applications will be discussed, though the technique is a valuable research tool. Ambulatory ECG monitoring has enabled the detection and diagnosis of intermittent disorders of cardiac rhythm thus elucidating the cause of symptoms such as syncope, palpitation and chest pain. The technique is most valuable when the patient actually experiences his usual symptoms during an ECG recording. The patient should be instructed to record the time of onset of his symptoms so that these can be correlated with the heart rhythm at that time. With some recorders the patient can operate an event marker which indicates the onset of symptoms on the tape. Even when the patient does not experience symptoms during recording, rhythm abnormalities of diagnostic significance may be detected. Obviously, if the patient does not experience symptoms during the recording and no rhythm abnormalities are found, an arrhythmic cause for the patient's symptoms cannot be excluded. Furthermore, in the absence of symptoms, the finding of a minor abnormality of rhythm does not exclude the possibility that the patient's complaints are due to a more major rhythm disturbance. It may be necessary to record several tapes before diagnostic information is obtained.

The technique has demonstrated that in patients with syncope but a normal routine ECG, sinus arrest is often, and complete AV block occasionally, the cause.

Ambulatory monitoring is of some value in assessing a patient's response to therapy. For example, not uncommonly a tape recording will reveal frequent ventricular arrhythmias in spite of the use of an anti-arrhythmic agent. One problem in using ambulatory monitoring to assess therapy is that there is a marked spontaneous variation in the frequency of arrhythmias and so on the basis of one tape, absence or improvement in arrhythmia may not necessarily be a consequence of drug therapy.

'Normal' findings

Sinus bradycardia, short pauses due to sino-atrial block and AV Wenkebach block can occur in normal people during sleep and should not be regarded as evidence of conduction tissue disease. These phenomena may also sometimes occur during the day in young people with high vagal tone.

Whereas a routine 12-lead electrocardiogram records approximately 60 heart beats, a normal 24-hour tape recording is likely to contain at least 90 000 beats. Thus ambulatory electrocardiography is a very much more sensitive tool than a standard recording. For example, the finding of a single ventricular ectopic beat on a routine ECG suggests a much higher frequency than a hundred ectopic beats on a 24-hour tape. In fact, studies of apparently normal people using ambulatory electrocardiography have shown that unifocal ventricular extrasystoles occur quite commonly, as do supraventricular ectopic beats. Some studies have also found very short runs of relatively slow ventricular tachycardia in apparently normal young subjects.

Artefacts

A number of technical problems during ambulatory electrocardiography can result in what appear to be arrhythmias to the unwary.

If the tape speed slows for any reason, complexes will appear closer together and mimic tachycardia. However, the duration of each ventricular complex will be shorter than normal and this should alert the observer to the likelihood of artefact. Conversely, if the tape runs too fast, apparent bradycardia with broader than normal complexes will result.

Not infrequently, a lead will become disconnected during a recording: since no activity is being recorded the ECG will appear as a straight line and mimic sinus arrest. Furthermore, sometimes an electrical connection can intermittently fail, resulting in repeated episodes of apparent sinus arrest. However, if a lead becomes disconnected it is likely to do so at any point in the cardiac cycle, and it is unlikely that the onset of 'asystole' will arise after the ventricular T wave as it would if sinus arrest were real. If the onset of sinus arrest does occur during the inscription of an atrial or ventricular complex, artefact can be assumed.

Occasionally, artefact can produce an apparent tachycardia but close inspection will reveal that normal QRS complexes are 'walking through' the tachycardia.

Infrequent palpitation

Patients with infrequent palpitation are unlikely to experience an episode during a 24-hour recording. Recently, a very useful and relatively inexpensive device (cardio-memo recorder) has been introduced which will record 30 s of electrocardiogram. The patient can carry the device around until an attack occurs. He or she then applies the device to the chest wall and activates the recording which is stored in a memory and can be replayed directly or via the telephone into an ECG machine.

Clearly, the device is not suitable for the investigation of episodes that disable the patient to the extent that they cannot activate the recorder. It is very important that it is explained to the patient precisely when and how to use the recorder.

Main points

♦ Ambulatory electrocardiography is very useful for the investigation of syncope, near-syncope, palpitation and other symptoms thought to be due to an arrhythmia when routine electrocardiography has not provided diagnostic information.

♦ Artefact can produce apparent arrhythmias but can usually be recognized by careful inspection of the recording.

♦ Studies in apparently normal subjects have demonstrated that certain rhythm disturbances detected by ambulatory electrocardiography are not of pathological significance.

♦ For patients with infrequent, non-disabling palpitation, provision of a cardio-memo recorder is the best method of investigation.

♦ Useful information will be provided from an ambulatory recording if an arrhythmia is demonstrated or if a patient experiences his usual symptoms without a disturbance in rhythm. Clearly if there is no arrhythmia and no symptoms, an episodic arrhythmia has not been excluded.

Chapter 18

Intracardiac electrophysiological testing

Information derived from intracardiac electrophysiological testing has led to an increased understanding of conduction defects and tachycardias.

In the assessment of the individual patient, the technique has a limited role. Its main uses are for investigating the feasibility of pacing techniques or surgery for control of tachyarrhythmias. In addition, it is occasionally valuable in detecting abnormal function of the sinus node or AV junction in patients with suspected conduction tissue disease in whom repeated standard and ambulatory electrocardiography has been uninformative. Similarly, in patients with infrequent palpitation in whom ambulatory electrocardiography has not provided diagnostic information, the technique can be used to try to initiate a tachycardia.

Here, discussion will be limited to a brief account of the technique and some of its uses.

Technique

The sequence of cardiac chamber activation, during normal and abnormal rhythms, is studied by recording electrograms from various intracardiac sites using transvenous bipolar electrodes which are introduced via femoral and antecubital veins under local anaesthesia.

Activity from the right atrium, left atrium, ventricles and bundle of His can be recorded by positioning electrodes in the right atrium, in the coronary sinus (which passes behind the left atrium), right ventricle and across the tricuspid valve, respectively. The intracardiac electrograms together with surface leads are recorded simultaneously on a multi-channel recorder, usually at a paper speed of 100 mm/s (Figure 18.1).

His bundle electrogram

Careful positioning of an electrode across the tricuspid valve enables His bundle activity to be recorded (Figure 18.1). Activity from the low right atrium and interventricular septum is also recorded. The three waves are designated H, A and V, respectively. The A–H interval indicates the time taken for an atrial impulse to be conducted through the AV node, and the H–V interval represents the time taken for transmission through the bundle of His and the bundle branches to the ventricles.

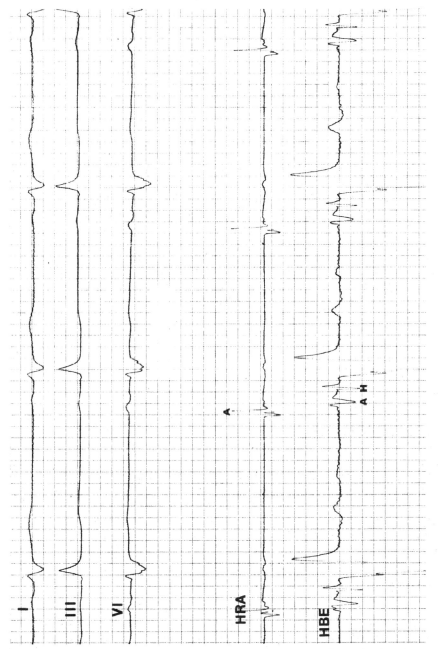

Figure 18.1 Simultaneous recording, at 100 mm/s, of surface leads I, III and V1 together with a high right atrial electrogram (HRA) and His bundle electrogram (HBE). A, atrial activity; H, His bundle activity

Pacing

The recording electrodes can also be used for atrial or ventricular stimulation. Two basic methods of pacing are employed: first, regular pacing at various rates; secondly, using a programmable stimulator, precisely timed premature stimuli can be introduced during spontaneous or paced rhythm (see Figure 18.4). These can be timed to occur progressively earlier in the cardiac cycle so that the whole cycle is scanned. Sometimes double or triple stimuli are used.

Clinical applications

AV conduction

In patients with complete heart block, knowledge of whether the block is at AV nodal or infranodal level may be of practical significance (see Chapter 9). In patients with AV nodal block the subsidiary pacemaker will be in the bundle of His and each ventricular complex will, therefore, be preceded by a His bundle spike (Figure 18.2). On the other hand, when the block is infranodal, His bundle and ventricular activity will be dissociated.

The normal H–V interval, which is a measure of conduction time through the bundle of His and bundle branches, is 35–55 ms. Any increase indicates impaired conduction.

In patients with bifascicular block a prolonged H–V interval is evidence of slowed conduction in the functioning fascicle and means that there is trifascicular disease (however, prophylactic pacing of patients with trifascicular disease is not of proven benefit).

Occasionally, in patients with infrequent Stokes–Adams attacks, it may not be possible to establish the cause in spite of standard and continuous ambulatory electrocardiograms. Prolongation of the H–V interval strongly points to abnormal AV conduction, though a normal measurement does not exclude impaired conduction. Sometimes H–V prolongation can only be induced when the intraventricular conducting system is stressed by an atrial ectopic beat (Figure 18.3).

Sick sinus syndrome

Intracardiac electrophysiological testing may be useful in patients in whom the sick sinus syndrome is suspected but cannot be proved by surface electrocardiography. In normal subjects cessation of rapid atrial pacing or single premature atrial stimuli leads to only a brief pause before sinus node activity resumes. In patients with sick sinus syndrome a profound depression of sinus node activity can result. When the 'sinus node recovery time' is greater than 140% of the sinus cycle length, sick sinus syndrome should be suspected. An extreme example is shown in Figure 18.4.

An atrial pacemaker can be used in cases of sick sinus syndrome only if AV function is satisfactory. If second-degree AV block develops at relatively low atrial pacing rates (e.g. less than 120/min) of if there is a prolonged H–V interval, atrial pacing is usually contraindicated.

Atrial activity during tachycardia

A right atrial electrogram can sometimes be of great diagnostic help when atrial

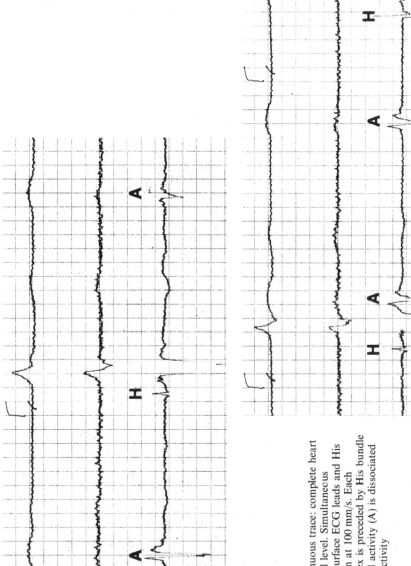

Figure 18.2 Continuous trace: complete heart block at AV nodal level. Simultaneous recording of two surface ECG leads and His bundle electrogram at 100 mm/s. Each ventricular complex is preceded by His bundle activity (H). Atrial activity (A) is dissociated from ventricular activity

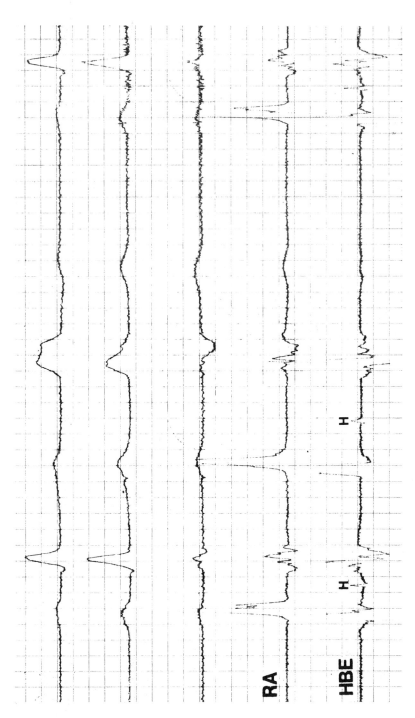

Figure 18.3 Simultaneous recordings of leads I, II and III together with right atrial electrogram (RA) and His bundle electrogram (HBE) at 100 mm/s. The second complex is an atrial ectopic beat conducted with left bundle branch block. In this beat, the H–V interval is markedly increased at 140 ms

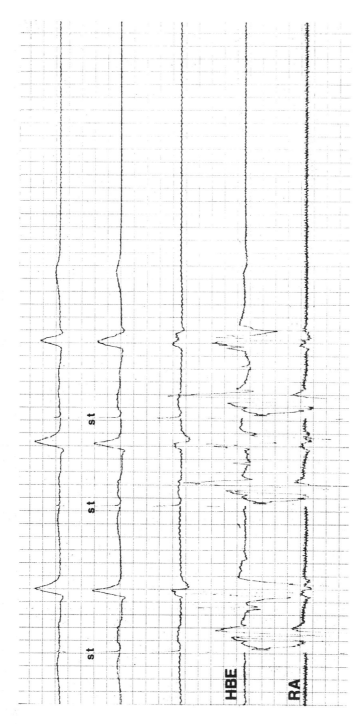

Figure 18.4 Simultaneous recording of three surface ECG leads together with His bundle (HBE) and right atrial (RA) electrograms at 100 mm/s. Right atrial pacing stimuli (st) at regular intervals of 570 ms are followed by a single extrastimulus with a coupling interval of 340 ms. This resulted in total cardiac standstill over 5 s after which the pacemaker had to be re-started. The premature atrial stimulus also slightly increased the duration of the H–V interval

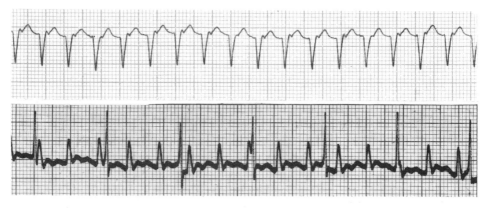

Figure 18.5 Recording at 25 mm/s of lead V5 and right atrial electrogram in a patient with acute anterior myocardial infarction thought to have had paroxysmal supraventricular tachycardia. Atrial activity is slower than and dissociated from the ventricular activity, indicating that the tachycardia is of His bundle or ventricular origin

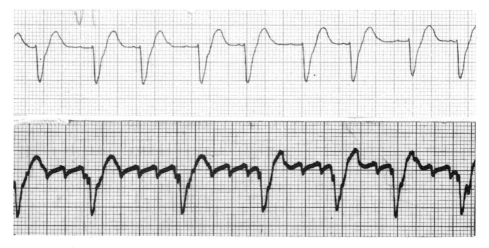

Figure 18.6 Recording of lead V1 and right atrial electrogram in a patient with a tachycardia and left bundle branch block. The atrial electrogram shows atrial flutter, although this was not clear from any of the surface ECG leads

activity during tachycardia cannot be identified from the surface electrocardiogram (Figures 18.5 and 18.6).

Paroxysmal supraventricular tachycardia

Paroxysmal supraventricular tachycardia can usually be initiated and terminated by precisely timed premature atrial or ventricular stimuli (Figures 18.7 and 18.8). The ability to stop and start tachycardias allows the effects of drugs and pacing techniques to be studied.

When surgery is being considered for paroxysmal supraventricular tachycardia it is important to know whether the re-entrant circuit is made up by a bundle of Kent

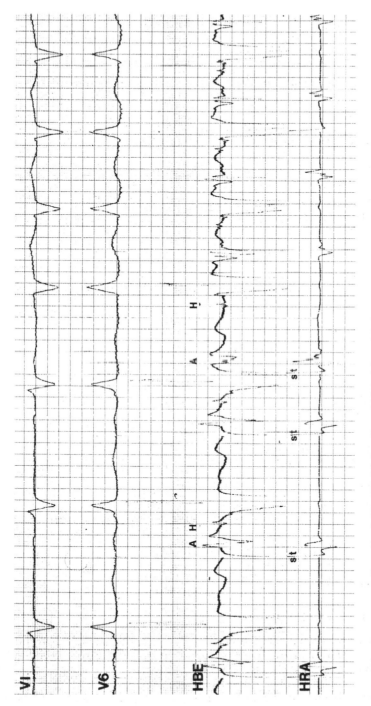

Figure 18.7 Simultaneous recording of leads V1, V6, His bundle and high right atrial electrograms at 100 mm/s. The right atrium is being stimulated (st) at intervals of 530 ms after which an atrial extra-stimulus with a coupling interval of 260 ms is introduced. The extra-stimulus initiates supraventricular tachycardia

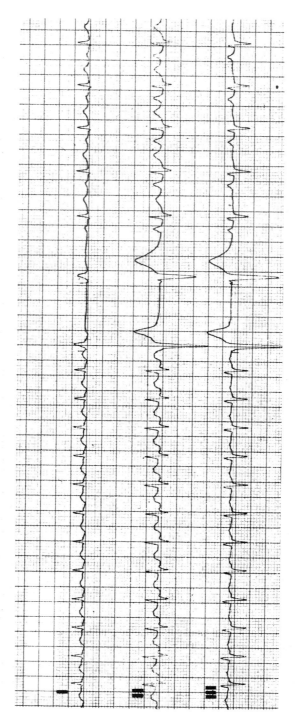

Figure 18.8 Paroxysmal supraventricular tachycardia terminated by the first of two paced ventricular beats

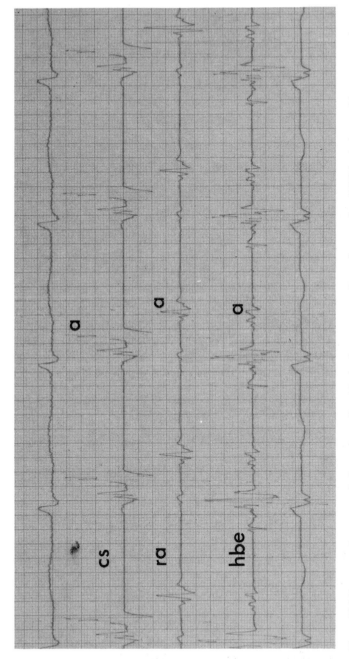

Figure 18.9 Paroxysmal supraventricular tachycardia with simultaneous recordings of two surface ECG leads (top and bottom traces) together with coronary sinus (**cs**), right atrial (**ra**) and His bundle (**hbe**) electrograms. Atrial activity (**a**) in the coronary sinus electrogram (which reflects the left atrial activity) precedes right atrial activity during the tachycardia, indicating that the re-entrant mechanism uses a left-sided bundle of Kent

or an additional intra-AV nodal pathway (see Chapter 6). Even in patients with the Wolff–Parkinson–White syndrome the tachycardia sometimes does not involve the bundle of Kent but is due to dual AV nodal pathways. Recording of the sequence of atrial activation during tachycardia usually allows distinction between the two mechanisms. In tachycardia due to dual AV nodal pathways, because the ventricular impulse re-enters the atria via the AV node, atrial activity will be first recorded by the His bundle electrode, since it is nearest to the AV node. On the other hand, if re-entry occurs via a left- or right-sided bundle of Kent, atrial activation will be recorded first in either coronary sinus or lateral right atrial electrograms. Many cases of paroxysmal supraventricular tachycardia without surface ECG evidence of pre-excitation have been shown to have a concealed left-sided bundle of Kent using this technique (Figure 18.9).

Atrial fibrillation in the Wolff–Parkinson–White syndrome

Atrial fibrillation in the Wolff–Parkinson–White syndrome can lead to a dangerously fast ventricular rate. The ventricular response to atrial fibrillation can be studied by inducing atrial fibrillation by rapid (250–1000 stimuli/min) atrial pacing. If the ventricular rate is dangerously fast, the procedure can be repeated after administration of a drug to ensure that the ventricular response is slowed (see Chapter 7).

Ventricular tachycardia

Sustained ventricular tachycardia may often be induced in patients who are prone to this arrhythmia by stimulating the heart with precisely timed single or double premature ventricular stimuli. Drug therapy which then prevents re-induction of the arrhythmia or at least increases the cycle length during tachycardia by over 100 ms has been shown to have a favourable effect on prognosis. Serial testing may be required to identify an effective drug. Sometimes all anti-arrhythmic drugs will be found to be ineffective.

There are reservations about the predictive value of electrophysiological testing. The more aggressive the stimulation protocol in terms of the number of stimuli and the rate of stimulation, the easier it is to induce a ventricular arrhythmia. It is not clear which stimulation protocol has the best predictive accuracy. There is doubt as to the significance of induction of non-sustained ventricular tachycardia. It does not necessarily follow that the oral preparation of a drug that has proved effective when given intravenously during an electrophysiological test will prevent spontaneous ventricular arrhythmias. Amiodarone may prevent spontaneous ventricular tachycardia and yet the arrhythmia may still be inducible, albeit usually at a relatively slow rate, at electrophysiological testing.

Chapter 19

Arrhythmias for interpretation: a quiz

In this chapter examples of a variety of arrhythmias are given. The 'answers' appear on pages 196–199. As is often the case in practice, there may be more than one observation to make about each example.

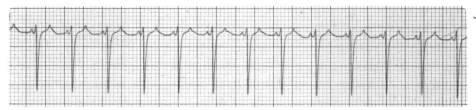

Figure 19.1 Lead V1

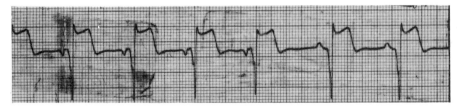

Figure 19.2 Lead AVF

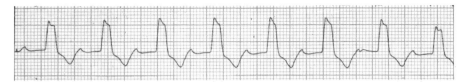

Figure 19.3 Lead I

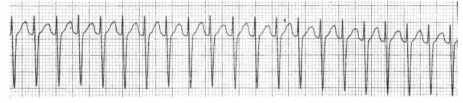

Figure 19.4

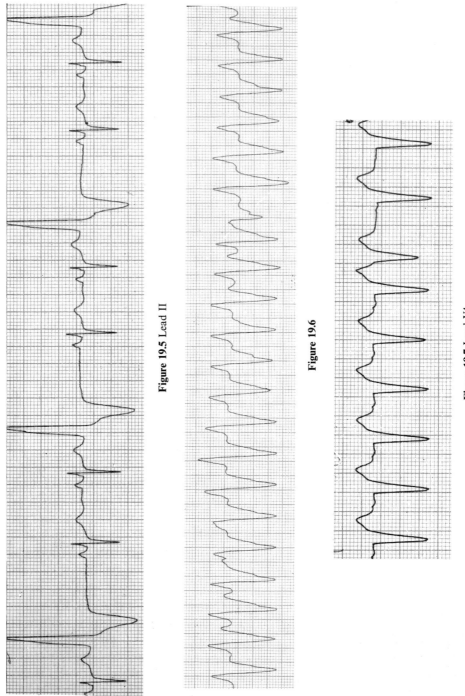

Figure 19.5 Lead II

Figure 19.6

Figure 19.7 Lead V1

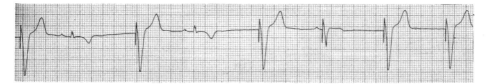

Figure 19.8 Lead II

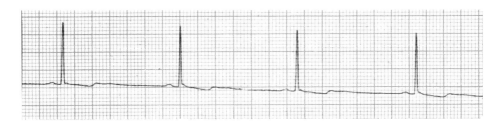

Figure 19.9

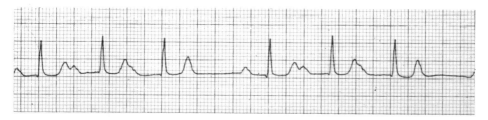

Figure 19.10 Lead AVF

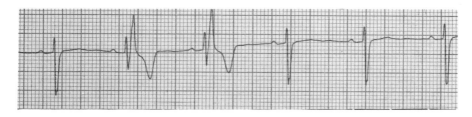

Figure 19.11 Lead V1

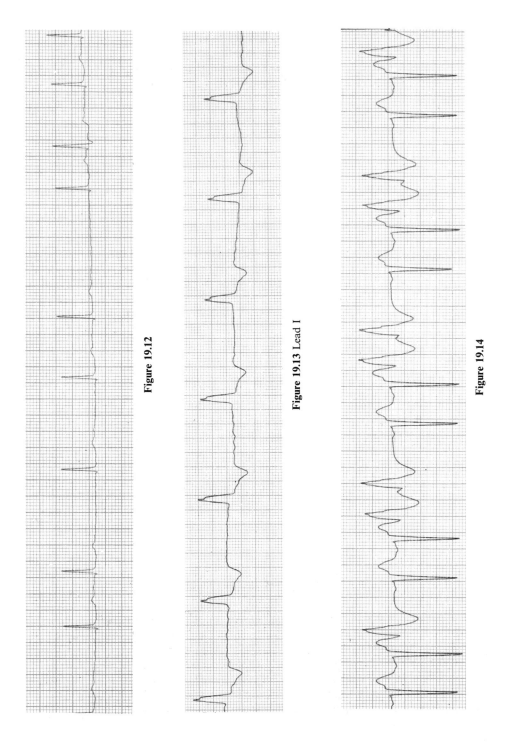

Figure 19.12

Figure 19.13 Lead I

Figure 19.14

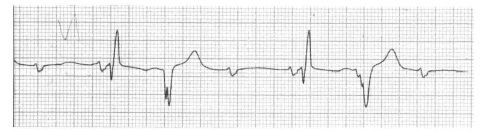

Figure 19.15 Lead V1

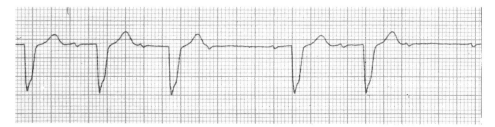

Figure 19.16 Lead AVF

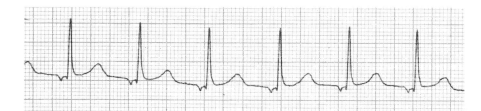

Figure 19.17 Lead V1

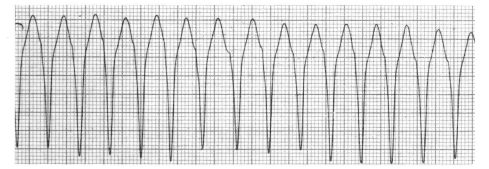

Figure 19.18

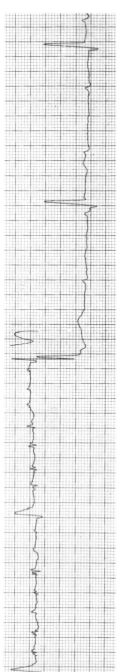

Figure 19.19 Continuous recording as lead is changed from AVR to V1

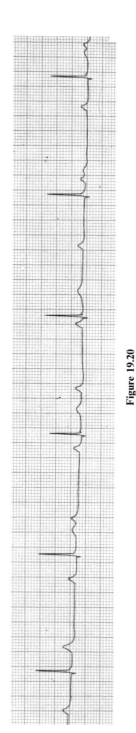

Figure 19.20

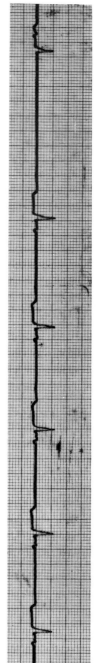

Figure 19.21

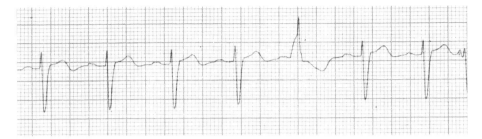

Figure 19.22

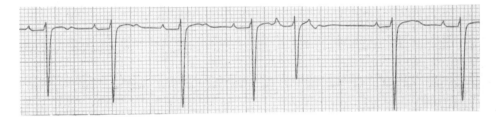

Figure 19.23

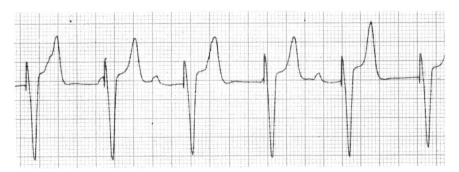

Figure 19.24 Lead II

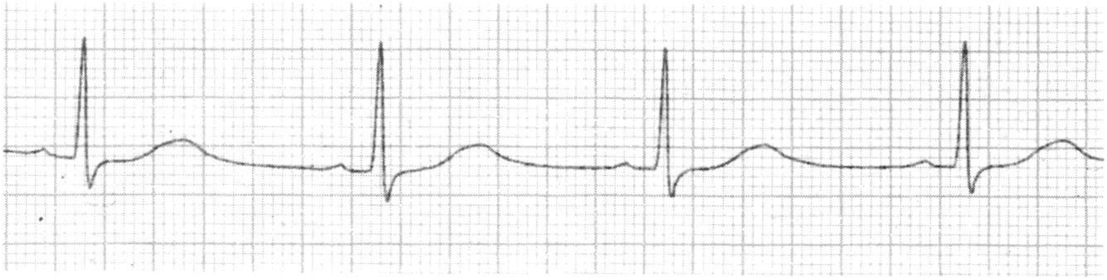

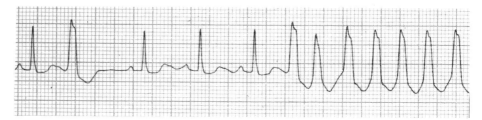

Figure 19.25 Lead I

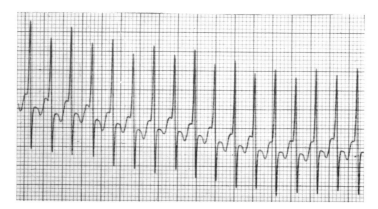

Figure 19.26

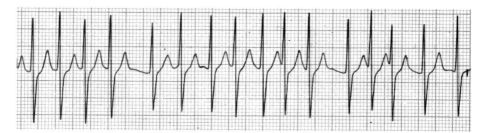

Figure 19.27

Figure 19.28

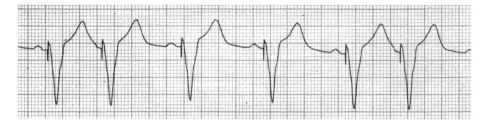

Figure 19.29 Lead II

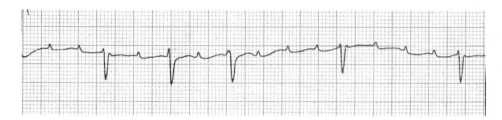

Figure 19.30 Lead V1

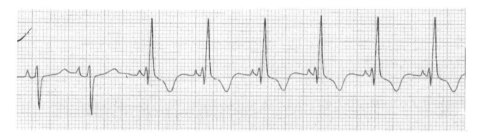

Figure 19.31 Lead V1

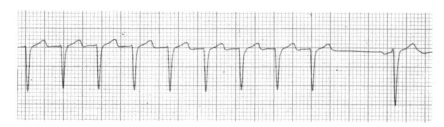

Figure 19.32 Lead V1

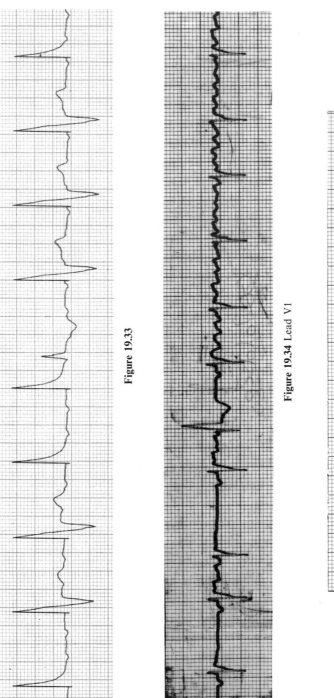

Figure 19.33

Figure 19.34 Lead V1

Figure 19.35

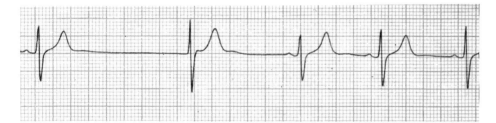

Figure 19.36

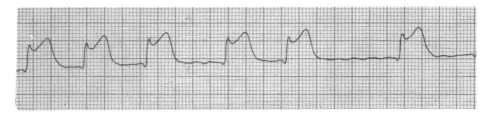

Figure 19.37 Lead AVF

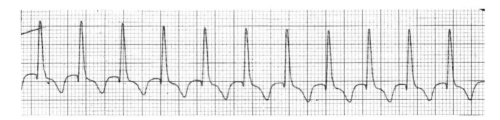

Figure 19.38

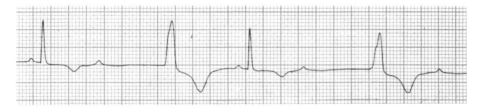

Figure 19.39

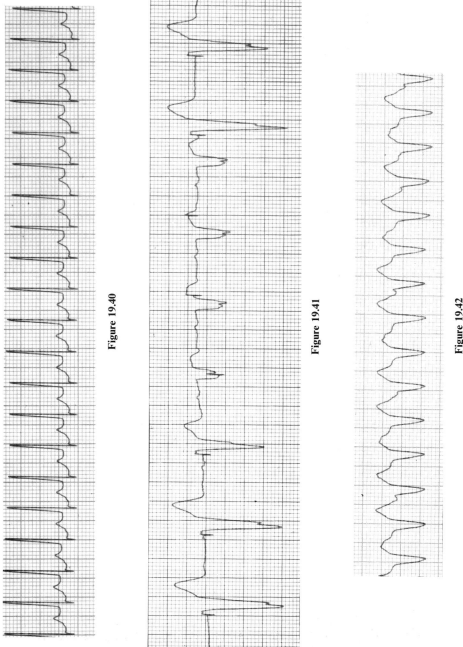

Figure 19.40

Figure 19.41

Figure 19.42

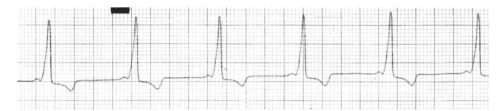

Figure 19.43 Lead V6

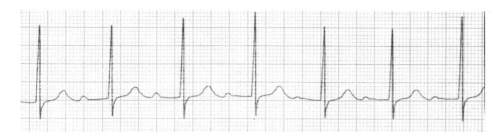

Figure 19.44

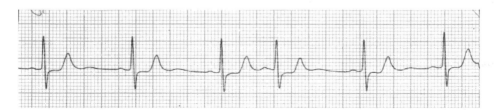

Figure 19.45

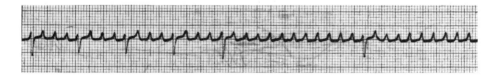

Figure 19.46

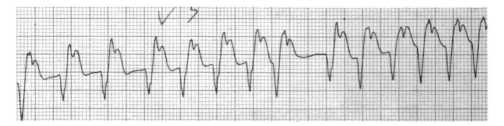

Figure 19.47 Lead V3

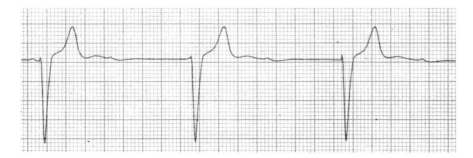

Figure 19.48

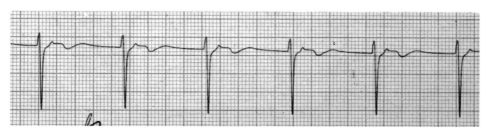

Figure 19.49

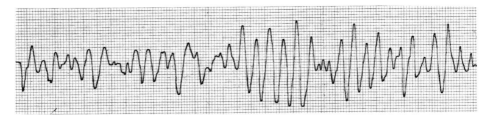

Figure 19.50

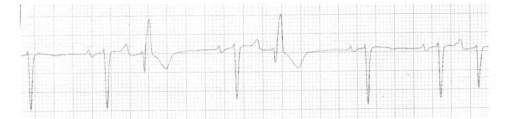

Figure 19.51 Lead V1

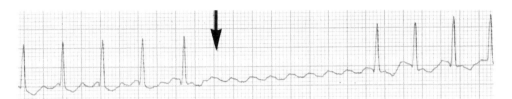

Figure 19.52 Arrow indicates carotid sinus massage

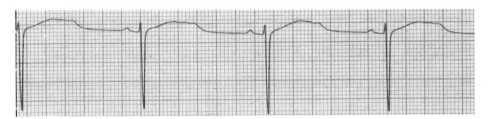

Figure 19.53

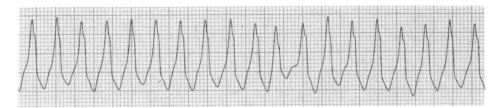

Figure 19.54

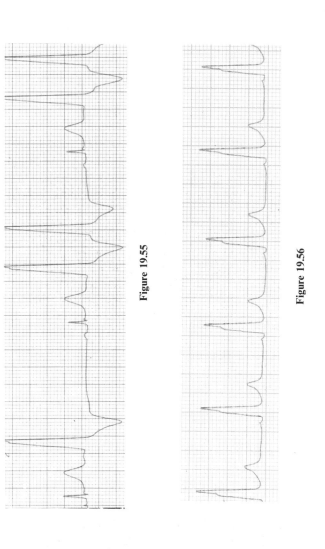

Figure 19.55

Figure 19.56

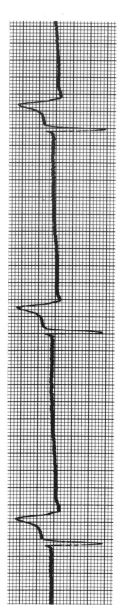

Figure 19.57

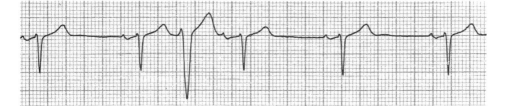

Figure 19.58

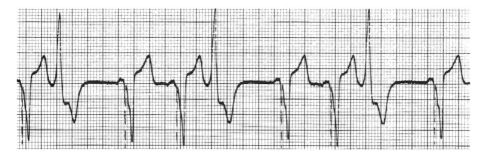

Figure 19.59

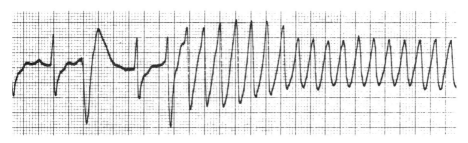

Figure 19.60

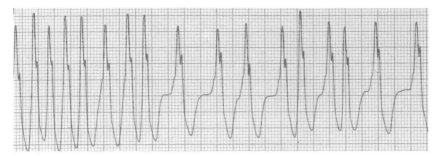

Figure 19.61

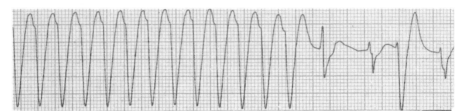

Figure 19.62

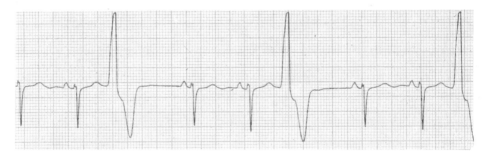

Figure 19.63

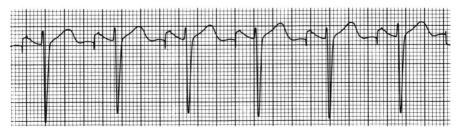

Figure 19.64

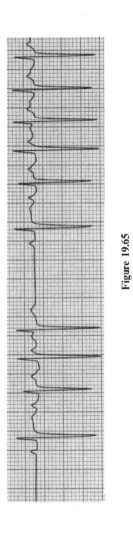

Figure 19.65

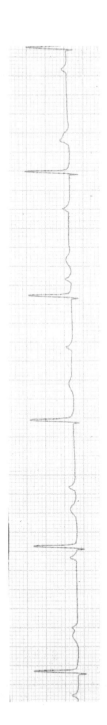

Figure 19.66

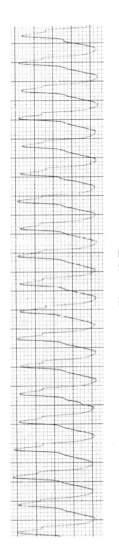

Figure 19.67

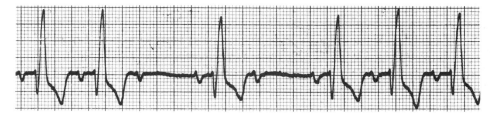

Figure 19.68

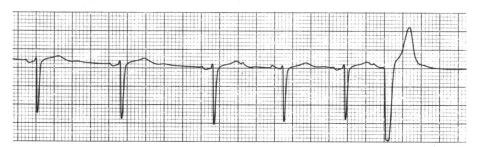

Figure 19.69

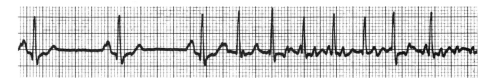

Figure 19.70

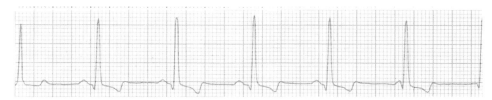

Figure 19.71

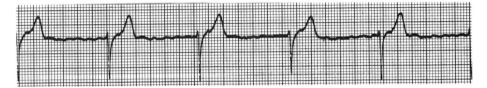

Figure 19.72

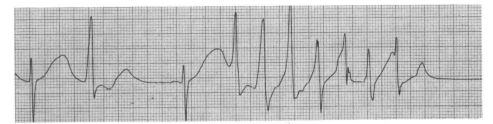

Figure 19.73

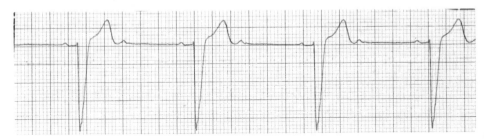

Figure 19.74

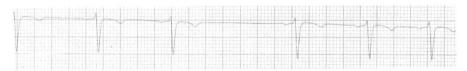

Figure 19.75

Answers

Figure 19.1. Atrial flutter with 2:1 AV block

Figure 19.2 Inferior myocardial infarction. The first five beats are of junctional origin

Figure 19.3 Left bundle branch block with first-degree AV block. A 'P' wave is superimposed on the end of the preceding T wave

Figure 19.4 Paroxysmal supraventricular tachycardia

Figure 19.5 Sinus rhythm with ventricular trigeminy. The ventricular complexes during sinus rhythm are predominantly negative, indicating left axis deviation

Figure 19.6 Ventricular tachycardia. The sixteenth beat is a fusion beat

Figure 19.7 Left bundle branch block as indicated by the broad QS complexes in lead V1. An atrial ectopic beat is superimposed on the T wave of the seventh beat and is also conducted with left bundle branch block

Figure 19.8 Ventricular demand pacemaker inhibited by sinus beats. The sixth complex is a fusion beat

Figure 19.9 Sinus bradycardia

Figure 19.10 AV Wenkebach phenomenon. The non-conducted beat is superimposed on the T wave of the preceding beat

Figure 19.11 Intermittent right bundle branch block

Figure 19.12 Atrial fibrillation with slow ventricular response

Figure 19.13 Atrial fibrillation with complete AV block

Figure 19.14 Single and coupled ventricular extrasystoles

Figure 19.15 2:1 AV block with ventricular ectopic beats

Figure 19.16 Junctional rhythm. Each ventriclar complex is preceded by an inverted P wave indicating that the junctional focus has also activated the atria

Figure 19.17 AV Wenkebach block with left bundle branch block

Figure 19.18 Ventricular tachycardia

Figure 19.19 V1 shows complete AV block. The apparent rapid atrial activity in lead AVR is caused by somatic tremor due to Parkinson's disease

Figure 19.20 Complete AV block with narrow ventricular complexes

Figure 19.21 Sinus bradycardia with sinus arrest followed by a junctional escape beat

Figure 19.22 Sinus rhythm with an end-diastolic ventricular ectopic beat

Figure 19.23 Atrial ectopic beat superimposed on fourth ventricular T wave

Figure 19.24 Ventricular pacing. Dissociated atrial activity can clearly be seen

Figure 19.25 Sinus bradycardia with prolonged QT interval (QTc = 0·53 s)

Figure 19.26 Tachycardia of supraventricular origin with a rate of 290/min suggesting atrial flutter with 1:1 AV conduction

Figure 19.27 The second ventricular ectopic beat initiates ventricular tachycardia

Figure 19.28 Atrial fibrillation with rapid ventricular response

Figure 19.29 Atrial synchronized pacing. After the first and fifth ventricular complexes there are atrial extrasystoles which also trigger ventricular pacing

Figure 19.30 Atrial tachycardia with variable AV conduction

Figure 19.31 Sinus rhythm. Last six beats conducted with right bundle branch block

Figure 19.32 Paroxysmal supraventricular tachycardia which terminates after the ninth beat

Figure 19.33 Intermittent failure to capure of ventricular demand pacemaker: first, fourth, fifth and ninth pacing stimuli fail to capture ventricles. After fifth stimulus, spontaneous ventricular beat inhibits pacemaker indicating satisfactory sensing. In addition, there is an atrial tachycardia

Figure 19.34 Atrial ectopic beats follow the second, fourth and sixth ventricular complexes. The first ectopic beat is conducted normally, the second with right bundle branch block and the third leads to atrial fibrillation

Figure 19.35 Complete AV block with broad ventricular complexes

Figure 19.36 Following the first sinus beat there is sinus arrest and a junctional escape beat

Figure 19.37 Acute inferior myocardial infarction and atrial fibrillation with slow ventricular response

Figure 19.38 Junctional tachycardia

Figure 19.39 Second-degree AV block with ventricular ectopic beats

Figure 19.40 Paroxysmal supraventricular tachycardia

Figure 19.41 Fixed rate ventricular pacing. The pacemaker is not inhibited by the period of sinus rhythm after the third paced beat

Figure 19.42 Ventricular tachycardia. There are peaks at regular intervals superimposed on the T waves of the first, fourth, seventh, tenth and thirteenth complexes which may be due to independent atrial activity

Figure 19.43 Sinus rhythm with Wolff–Parkinson–White syndrome

Figure 19.44 First-degree AV block. PR interval = 0·30 s

Figure 19.45 After the third sinus beat there is an atrial ectopic beat

Figure 19.46 Atrial flutter conducted with varying degrees of AV block

Figure 19.47 Atrial fibrillation in acute anterior myocardial infarction

Figure 19.48 Complete AV block. The third and fifth atrial impulses are concealed by ventricular complexes

Figure 19.49 Junctional rhythm with retrograde atrial conduction

Figure 19.50 Ventricular fibrillation

Figure 19.51 Atrial ectopic beats superimposed on ventricular T waves of second, fourth and sixth ventricular complexes. The first two are conducted with right bundle branch block

Figure 19.52 Atrial flutter with 2:1 AV block. Carotid massage causes transient complete AV block

Figure 19.53 Sinus rhythm with long QT interval and prominent U waves (due to amiodarone)

Figure 19.54 Ventricular tachycardia with capture beat

Figure 19.55 Ventricular ectopic beats including couplets after second and third sinus beats

Figure 19.56 Sinus rhythm with Wolff–Parkinson–White syndrome

Figure 19.57 Sinus arrest. Ventricular escape rhythm

Figure 19.58 Interpolated ventricular ectopic beat with retrograde concealed ventriculo-atrial conduction

Figure 19.59 Atrial synchronized ventricular pacing. Two ventricular extrasystoles inhibit universal (DDD) pacemaker

Figure 19.60 Second ventricular ectopic beat initiates ventricular flutter/fibrillation

Figure 19.61 Atrial fibrillation. QRS morphology suggests delta waves, i.e. Wolff–Parkinson–White syndrome

Figure 19.62 Paroxysmal supraventricular tachycardia

Figure 19.63 Ventricular trigeminy

Figure 19.64 Atrial pacing

Figure 19.65 Paroxysmal atrial tachycardia

Figure 19.66 Complete AV block

Figure 19.67 Ventricular tachycardia

Figure 19.68 Intermittent Mobitz II AV block

Figure 19.69 Atrial ectopic beats superimposed on third and fifth ventricular T waves. First ectopic is not conducted, the second is conducted to the ventricles with left bundle branch block

Figure 19.70 Paroxysmal atrial fibrillation

Figure 19.71 AV dissociation

Figure 19.72 Atrial fibrillation with complete AV block

Figure 19.73 Sinus bradycardia with marked QT prolongation and short run of torsade de pointes tachycardia

Figure 19.74 2:1 AV block. Conducted beats show left bundle branch block

Figure 19.75 2:1 sino-atrial block

Index